CW00321782

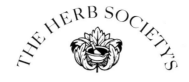

THE HERB SOCIETY'S

HOME HERBAL

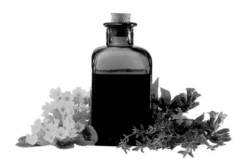

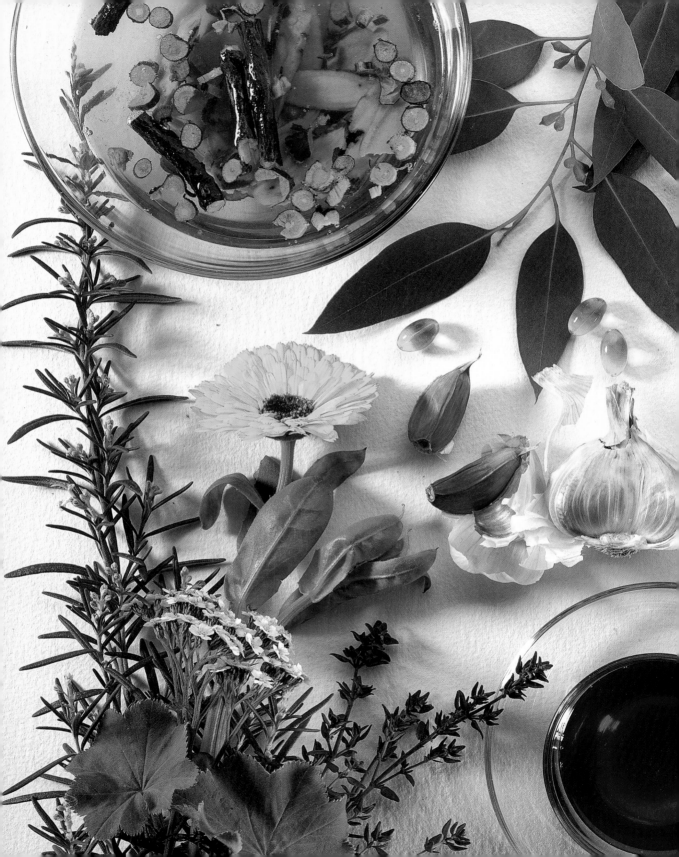

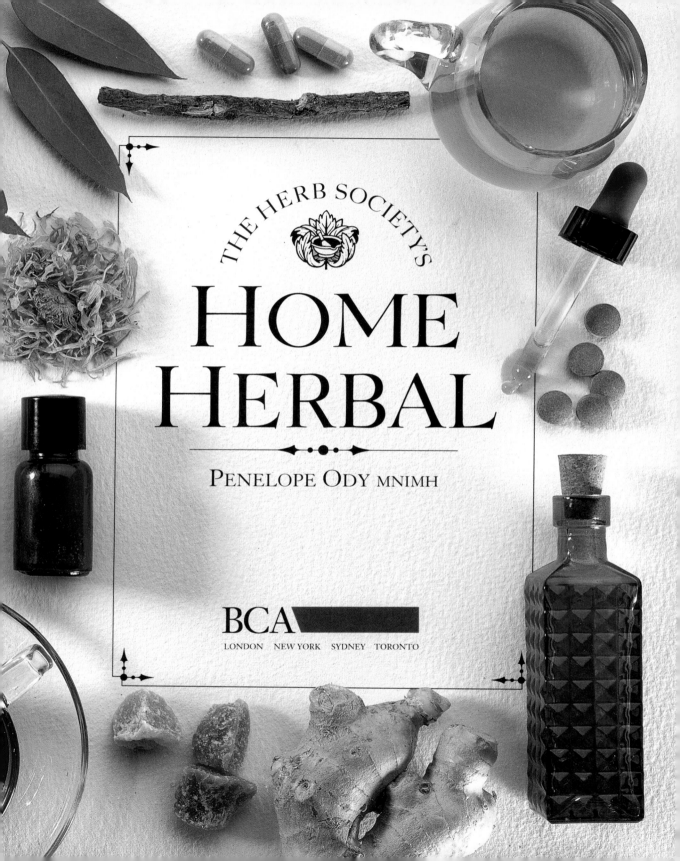

THE HERB SOCIETY'S

HOME
HERBAL

PENELOPE ODY MNIMH

BCA

LONDON NEW YORK SYDNEY TORONTO

A DORLING KINDERSLEY BOOK

Art Editor Jane Bull   Project Editor Penny Warren
Managing Editor Rosie Pearson   Senior Managing Art Editor Carole Ash
DTP Designer Karen Ruane   Production Manager Maryann Rogers

In memory of my father
S. M. Ody
1915–1994
with love and thanks

IMPORTANT NOTICE

The recommendations and information in this book are appropriate in most
cases. The advice this book contains is general, not specific to individuals and
their particular circumstances. Any plant substance, whether used as food or
medicine, externally or internally, can cause an allergic reaction in some people.
Neither the author nor the publishers can be held responsible for any injury,
damage or otherwise resulting from the use of herbal medicines. Do not try self-
diagnosis or attempt self-treatment for serious or long-term problems without
consulting a medical professional or qualified practitioner. Do not undertake any
self-treatment while you are undergoing a prescribed course of medical
treatment without first seeking professional advice. Always seek medical advice
if symptoms persist. Do not take essential oils internally except under
professional direction. Do not exceed any dosages recommended without
professional guidance. The use of some herbs is contraindicated in pregnancy or
in certain conditions. Check the list of herbs to avoid in pregnancy on p. 126 and
check the cautions in *A-to-Z of Medicinal Herbs* pp. 30–47 and *Other Medicinal
Herbs* pp. 138–40. See also *Essential Information* on p. 83.

This edition published 1995
by BCA by arrangement with
Dorling Kindersley Limited,
9 Henrietta Street, London WC2E 8PS

CN 5703

Copyright © 1995 Dorling Kindersley Limited, London
Text copyright © 1995 Penelope Ody

All rights reserved. No part of this publication may be reproduced, stored in a
retrieval system, or transmitted in any form or by any means, electronic,
mechanical, photocopying, recording or otherwise, without the prior written
permission of the copyright owner.

A CIP catalogue record for this book is available from the British Library

ISBN 0 7513 0166 3

Reproduced in Singapore by Colourscan
Printed and bound in Italy by New Interlitho, Milan

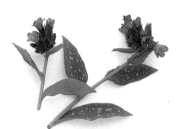

CONTENTS

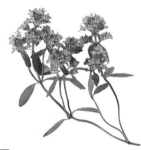

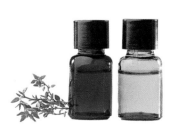

INTRODUCTION

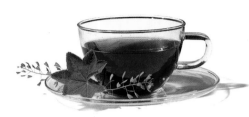

DESPITE the advances of modern medicine, the vast majority of the world's population still depends on herbal remedies to cure its ills. In some parts of the world, these remedies may be prescribed by a village medicine man (or woman) or by a local shaman. In other places, such as China and India, there are centuries-old, formal traditions of skilled herbal healing to call on. In the West, until the 1930s most medicines dispensed in high-street pharmacies were herbal and in many parts of Europe they are still the norm.

While major illnesses have always been referred to specialist healers, minor self-limiting ailments have traditionally been treated within the family, using remedies passed down through generations, much as favourite recipes for Christmas cake or winter soups are still handed down today. Every housewife had a repertoire of cure-alls to treat the family's ills. As well as a rather potent cough cure, my grandmother's favourites included the heart of an onion for earache and a well-worn left sock tied around the neck for sore throats! Some of these traditional medicines were based on what is now recognized as scientific fact, while others had more in common with faith-healing, but it was only if these household remedies failed that more sophisticated and expensive solutions were sought from the professionals. Illness, especially minor illness, was treated by and large within the family circle.

Today, life is very different. We have come to expect the quick "magic bullet" approach of modern medicine. Even common self-limiting ailments often warrant a trip to the general practitioner to be treated, in many cases, with unnecessarily powerful drugs that bring an assortment of side-effects. Ailments are treated superficially and symptomatically so that when the patient stops taking the medicine, the problem all too often returns. Infections may respond dramatically to antibiotics, but if they are the result of over-exhaustion and a weakened constitution, no amount of antibiotics will provide a permanent solution.

What is missing from the modern attitude to health is the sense that we are responsible for our own well-being. Many minor ailments are often of our own making, brought about by poor diet, lack of exercise or "burning the candle at both ends". Modern drugs may effect rapid apparent cures, but they cannot solve the problems we persistently bring on ourselves.

The approach of herbal medicine is not just about alleviating symptoms. More importantly, it is concerned with helping the body to cure itself. It is less magic bullet, more part of a balanced approach to living well. There is nothing inherently difficult about making and using herbal remedies, it is just that most of us in the developed world have lost the skills our grand-mothers and great-grandmothers took for granted. We have abandoned the basic folk wisdom of generations in favour of synthetic drugs that may not always stand the test of time.

In this book, I have suggested simple remedies for a variety of common ailments. It is not intended as a definitive guide, simply a range of practical suggestions that can be adapted, with experience, to suit the individual. The most important first step is to accept that good health lies in our own hands, and that, by being sensitive to our internal balance, we can often cure minor ills before they become major problems.

Penelope Ody

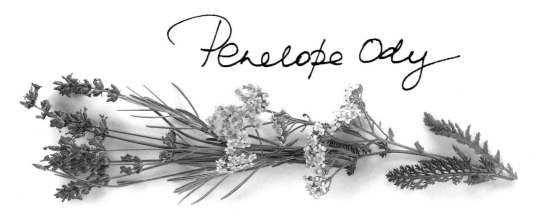

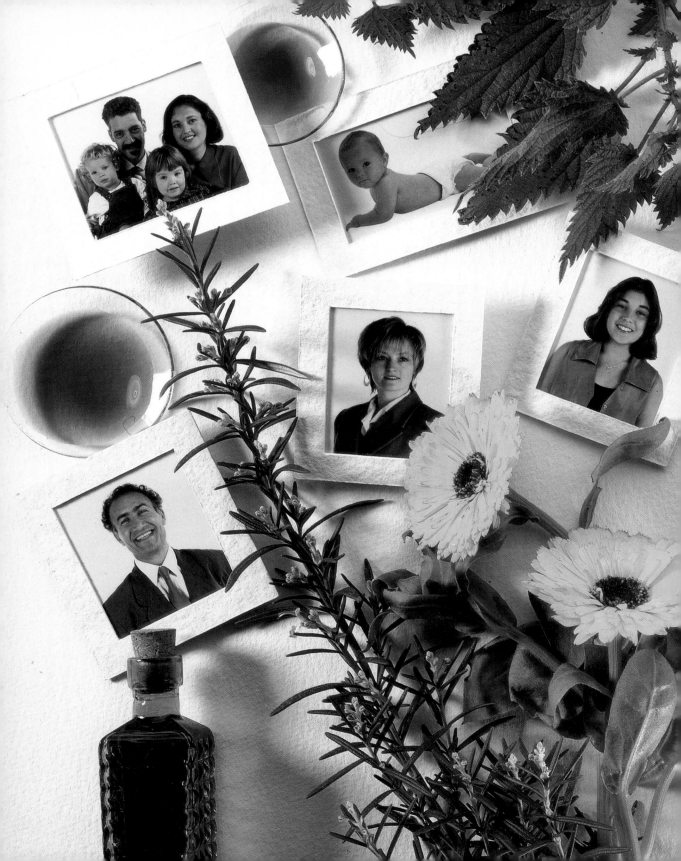

THE SEVEN LIFE STAGES

SHAKESPEARE DESCRIBED the seven ages of man in the 16th century and traditionally, each age, or life stage, has been seen as having distinct strengths and weaknesses, special energy requirements and particular problems. Today, the borderlines between the seven life stages have become blurred: the "newly retired" label, for example, can apply to people in their 50s and in their 70s. This section includes remedies, tonics and prophylactics that are especially suitable for each life stage. (The remedies can be taken individually or in combination.)

BABIES & TODDLERS

THE FIRST LIFE STAGE

WE LEARN AND grow more quickly during the first two years of life than at any other time. Small children have far more vital energy than most adults and can often prove a demanding and tireless handful. Babies and toddlers frequently become ill in a dramatic fashion. A child's metabolism is

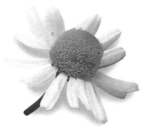

Chamomile flower

much faster than an adult's, with quicker heartbeat and breathing rates, and a fever will send his or her temperature soaring, before subsiding just as rapidly. Herbs can be very helpful for babies and toddlers, especially if they are introduced to them early, so that they become accustomed to the taste.

Preventative Treatments

Caution: Take professional advice if symptoms persist for more than 2–3 days. Do not give supplements for more than 2–3 weeks without taking professional advice. For dosage advice on remedies, vitamins and minerals, see p. 83. To make remedies, see pp. 62–79.

HERBS

CHAMOMILE is very soothing Put a couple of drops of oil in the bathwater at night, or give 25 ml of a weak infusion (use 10 g dried herb to 500 ml water).

EVENING PRIMROSE OIL contains essential fatty acids – lack of these chemicals can contribute to hyper-activity. Give 10–20 drops of oil on the tongue daily. This is not suitable for babies under 3 months.

HYSSOP helps chest problems by clearing excess mucus. Give half a cup (75 ml) of an infusion 2–3 times a week. Use 10 g dried herb to 500 ml water. Do not give to babies under 3 months and see Caution above.

VITAMINS & MINERALS

VITAMIN C should be taken in the form of fresh fruit and vegetables. If a child refuses to eat them, however, try giving flavoured vitamin C drinks.

IRON deficiency can result in learning difficulties. Guard against it with iron-rich foods, such as whole-meal bread, green vegetables, pulses, meat and eggs.

ZINC AND MANGANESE deficiencies can lead to sleep-lessness and hyperactivity. Supplements can help. Give a daily supplement containing 10 mg of zinc and 0.5–1 mg of manganese. Do not give to babies under 3 months and see Caution above.

GIVING HERBAL MEDICINES TO BABIES & TODDLERS

BITTER-TASTING HERBS
Sprinkle the powdered herb on bread spread with peanut butter, yeast extract, or other food that the child likes.

Herbs in peanut butter

SEEDS
Breakfast cereal is a useful camouflage for psyllium and other seeds. Mix them into cereal before adding milk.

Porridge with seeds

TINCTURES
Dilute the dose in a little warm water and, using a pipette, make a game of squirting drops on to the child's tongue.

Tincture and pipette

INFUSIONS
Blackcurrant or cranberry juice is useful to disguise infusions or tinctures. Add some pasteurized honey if constipation is a problem.

Infusion in blackcurrant juice

Health Profile

NEW FOODS, NEW EXPERIENCES, new infections – the young child has so much to cope with all at once that it is not surprising when occasional health problems arise. Although babies are born with the basis of a strong immune system, boosted by antibodies in the mother's milk, they can find it difficult to cope with polluting chemicals and bacteria, and are therefore vulnerable to infection. The remedies suggested may be taken individually or in combination. See Caution on p. 10.

TEETHING
Teething is a necessary, but unpleasant, aspect of babyhood.

Remedies
- *Chamomile or lemon balm infusion is soothing. Use 10 g dried herb to 500 ml water and give up to half a cup 3–6 times a day.*
- *Mix a teaspoon of slippery elm with a little water to make a paste and gently rub on the gums.*

SLEEPLESSNESS
Sleepless babies and young children upset the entire household as well as themselves. Make sure the child is comfortable, not too hot or cold, not hungry or thirsty, and that no insecurities or fears are causing the problem. Give plenty of cuddles.

Remedies
- *Add 500 ml of standard chamomile infusion or 2–3 drops of chamomile oil to bathwater at night to encourage sleep.*
- *Californian poppies are a gentle remedy for children. Give up to half a cup of weak infusion at night, made from 10 g dried herb to 500 ml water.*

HYPERACTIVITY

If a child is considerably more active than her contemporaries, it is worth checking the diet.

Remedies
- *Control food intake, avoiding synthetic additives and sugar.*
- *Give up to half a cup of weak agrimony and self-heal tea with a little pasteurized honey daily. Make the tea with 10 g dried herb and 500 ml water.*

COLIC
Rushed feeding may cause distressing spasms of the immature intestine.

Remedies
- *Make feeding the baby a relaxed process. If breastfeeding, drink weak dill, anise, fennel or catmint tea 3 times a day.*
- *Give 5 drops homeopathic chamomile (Chamomilla 3x) in a little water 3–4 times a day.*

RASHES AND ECZEMA
Rashes may look worse than they really are. Eczema can be related to food allergies.

Remedies
- *Bathe nappy rash in heartsease infusion and apply pot marigold ointment.*
- *To ease itching, apply a lotion made with 50 ml each of nettle juice and distilled witch hazel with 5 drops of rosemary oil.*

EARACHE
Childhood earache often starts at weaning and can recur. Milk allergy is a common cause.

Remedies
- *Use soya milk formulations instead of cow's milk.*
- *Put a little infused mullein oil in the ear and cover with a cottonwool swab. (Do not put anything in the ear if the drum is perforated.)*

CHILDREN

THE SECOND LIFE STAGE

FILLED WITH ENERGY, fun and laughter, childhood is ideally a time for carefree play, discovery, joy and learning. Of course, it is not always quite like that – children, too, experience tension and stress from sources such as school exams, family break-up or bullying. At such times, mild herbal tonics and relaxing mixtures can be extremely

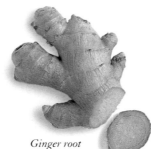

Ginger root

helpful. On the whole, children are remarkably healthy, and ailments are likely to be mild and self-limiting. In the developed world, at least, few children face life-threatening disorders. Herbs are ideal to treat children's ailments, although persuading them to take bitter-tasting remedies is not always easy (see p. 10).

Preventative Treatments

Caution: Take professional advice if symptoms persist for more than 2–3 days. Do not give supplements for more than 2–3 weeks without taking professional advice. For dosage advice on remedies, vitamins and minerals see p. 83. To make remedies, see pp. 62–79.

HERBS

GINGER is a pleasant-tasting herb, useful for combating travel sickness. It provides a warming remedy for colds and chills, and is soothing for digestive upsets. Give in the form of crystallized ginger or ginger biscuits as an alternative to ginger capsules.

LIQUORICE is helpful for constipation, a valuable tonic and children usually like its sweet taste. Give 10 drops of fluid extract up to 3 times a day.

SESAME SEEDS are rich in calcium and other minerals and provide a nutritious addition to the diet. Use them in cooking, on salads and with breakfast cereals.

VITAMINS & MINERALS

MAGNESIUM deficiency can cause muscle cramps, poor appetite, sleeplessness and behavioural problems. Give a daily supplement containing up to 800 mg.

ZINC deficiency is common in childhood and has been implicated in a wide range of problems, including dyslexia, growth problems, leg pains and insomnia. Give a daily supplement containing up to 50 mg.

B VITAMIN deficiencies, especially B¹ and B⁶, can lead to restlessness, fatigue and learning difficulties. Make sure the child is eating a healthy diet and give a daily supplement containing 10–20 mg of B¹ and 1–2mg of B⁶.

TIMELY TONICS

AMERICAN GINSENG
A gentle, but strengthening tonic, this suits children exhausted at the end of term or worn down by infections. Give 10 drops of tincture in a little warm water daily.

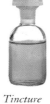

Tincture

SHU DI HUANG
A traditional Chinese childhood tonic, this herb strengthens growing bones and tissues. Give 10 drops of tincture in a little warm water daily.

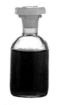

Tincture

GOTU KOLA
This Indian herb can be helpful for hyperactive children. Give a daily cup of infusion made with 15 g dried herb to 500 ml water.

Dried herb

SESAME OIL
Massage with warm sesame oil helps emotional upsets. Add 4 drops of lavender oil to 10 ml sesame oil and gently massage the shoulders and abdomen.

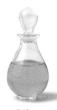

Oil

Health Profile

SCHOOL IS NOT JUST the place where children learn, it is also where they pick up infections and infestations, such as chickenpox, colds and head lice. Keeping children healthy, by ensuring they eat well and take plenty of fresh air, can help them combat such attacks. It also helps to limit their reliance on antibiotics, thereby avoiding immune system problems in later life.

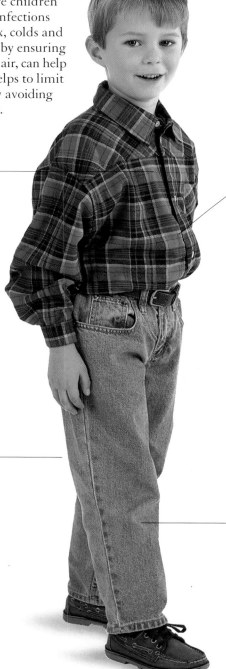

COLDS AND INFECTIONS
All day in an airless classroom, followed by hours playing computer games, is a sure way to encourage catarrh, stuffy heads and infections. Children's immune systems are usually strong, but recurring colds and repeated use of antibiotics soon weaken them.

Remedies
• *Give a cup of catmint infusion made with 20 g dried herb to 500 ml water, flavoured with a little honey or peppermint essence to help combat chills and catarrh.*
• *Give 10–20 drops of echinacea tincture in fruit juice daily to boost the immune system and combat infection.*

BEDWETTING
Anxiety, infections and inherited tendencies can all cause bedwetting. Lots of cuddles and affection may be needed if the problem is related to insecurity, such as from changing schools or moving house.

Remedies
• *Give 5–10 drops of sweet sumach or St John's wort tincture in warm water about 20 minutes before bed.*
• *For infections or bladder irritations, give a cup of buchu and cornsilk tea, made with 5 g of each dried herb and 200 ml water, 90 minutes before bedtime. Flavour with blackcurrant juice if desired.*

NITS
Head lice are common in schools. Check for eggs on the scalp, particularly at the nape of the neck.

Remedies
• *Put tea tree oil on a fine-toothed comb and comb the hair thoroughly weekly until the problem clears.*
• *Add 5 ml each of thyme and tea tree oils to 250 ml ordinary shampoo. Use to wash hair 2–3 times a week.*

UPSET TUMMIES AND DIARRHOEA
Excitement, over-eating, tension and antibiotics can all lead to digestive upsets or diarrhoea. Biliousness – attacks of nausea and vomiting – in childhood can be a forerunner of migraine in later life and may be linked to food sensitivities.

Remedies
• *Give plenty of fluids for diarrhoea – try blackcurrant or cranberry juice.*
• *For nausea and chronic diarrhoea, give a cup of ginger root decoction, (use 20 g root to 600 ml water).*
• *Give a runny paste made with 2 teaspoons of powdered slippery elm in hot water to soothe the stomach. Add yogurt to make it more palatable.*
• *For problems related to over-excitement, stress or food sensitivity, give a cup of lemon balm and agrimony tea made with 10 g of each dried herb to 500 ml water.*

CUTS AND GRAZES
Cuts and grazes are an inevitable part of childhood. Keep them clean and discourage children from picking the scabs.

Remedies
• *Add 5 ml of pot marigold tincture to 500 ml boiled water and bathe grazes from the centre outwards before applying a dressing or plaster.*
• *Use pot marigold or St John's wort cream on cuts and broken skin.*

ADOLESCENTS

THE THIRD LIFE STAGE

FOR BOTH SEXES, adolescence is a time of rapid physical and mental change. It is also an age for establishing self-confidence and forging a new adult identity. For some, this means a period of difficult and rebellious behaviour that may cause discord within the family. Testing the waters of adulthood usually involves experimentation – ranging

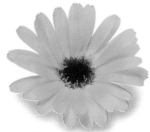
Pot marigold flower

from changing hairstyles, to smoking, drinking too much alcohol, having sex and abusing drugs. Luckily, most adolescents survive this life stage unscathed, and emerge, a little wiser, into young adulthood. Helpful remedies include Bach Flower Remedies to ease mood swings and tonics such as dandelion that cleanse the system.

Preventative Treatments

A healthy diet should be sufficient, but the following supplements may be useful during the growth spurts of adolescence.
For dosage advice on remedies, vitamins and minerals, see p. 83. For instructions on making remedies, see pp. 62–79.

HERBS

POT MARIGOLD is antifungal and antiseptic. Rub the cream regularly on to the face to help prevent spots.

ALFALFA is an excellent source of vitamins and minerals, which are often missing from the junk-food loved by teenagers. Use the sprouted seeds in sandwiches or as a garnish for omelettes and burgers.

DANDELION is a good liver tonic and cleansing herb, important for anyone exposed to synthetic chemicals, including food additives or those found in a polluted atmosphere. Take dandelion root as a decoction or use proprietary dandelion root coffee substitutes.

VITAMINS & MINERALS

CALCIUM is found in dairy products, green vegetables, nuts, seeds and pulses, and a healthy diet usually ensures an adequate supply. Calcium requirements are higher during growth periods so try eating more of these foods or take up to 250 mg daily.

ZINC is important for hormonal development. Boost intake by eating more meat, nuts, egg yolk, pulses and pumpkin seeds, or take up to 50 mg daily.

VITAMIN B[2] (riboflavin) requirements increase at times of rapid growth. Eat plenty of dairy produce, cereals and meat, or take 5–20 mg daily.

TIMELY TONICS

ROSEMARY
A stimulant tonic traditionally believed to improve the memory. Take a cup of standard infusion daily to improve concentration.
Fresh herb

CINNAMON
A warming tonic that is helpful during the hormonal changes and growth spurts of puberty. Try sprinkling the powder on hot buttered toast.
Cinnamon on toast

STINGING NETTLE
An ideal nutritional boost for a junk-food diet. Take 3 x 200 mg capsules or 10 ml juice daily.

BAI ZHI
To regulate the appetite, take 20 drops of tincture in warm water daily. For anorexia, mix with an equal amount of Chen Pi *and take 2 x 200 mg capsules 3 times daily.*

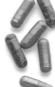
Capsules

Capsules

Health Profile

IRREGULAR MEALS, alcohol, late nights: the adolescent is almost asking for problems. Luckily, most teenagers remain extremely healthy, although burning the candle at both ends leads to increased risk of infection and glandular fever. Others may become obsessed with dieting and succumb to eating disorders such as anorexia.

GLANDULAR FEVER

Glandular fever occurs most commonly among adolescents and young adults. It usually starts with a sore throat, listlessness and aching muscles. Enlarged and tender glands can persist for up to 4 months.

Remedies
• *During the acute, early stages, take 5–10 ml each of echinacea and cleavers tinctures 3–4 times a day.*
• *During convalescence, mix equal amounts of Siberian ginseng, oats and vervain tinctures, and take 5 ml 4 times daily. Add a couple of drops of wormwood tincture to improve the appetite and aid digestion.*

MOODINESS AND IRRITABILITY

Mood swings, ranging from euphoria to depression and tears, are commonplace, as teenagers cope with the trials and tribulations of growing up.

Remedies
• *Bach Flower Remedies can be especially helpful: try vervain for feelings of injustice, and holly to combat anger and hatred. Take 9 drops of each diluted in 20 ml of water at frequent intervals.*
• *Add 2–3 drops of sandalwood and lavender oil to bathwater at night to aid relaxation.*

ACNE

Teenage spots can become a major preoccupation. The cause is likely to be poor diet and in girls they can be linked to menstrual irregularities, becoming worse before a period.

Remedies
• *Rubbing a garlic clove on spots at night or washing in water in which cabbage has been boiled, may not sound appealing, but both are effective treatments.*
• *Make a lotion with 30 ml each of pot marigold tincture, distilled witch hazel and rosewater with 5 ml of tea tree oil. Apply on some cottonwool 2–3 times daily.*

IRREGULAR OR PAINFUL PERIODS

It often takes 2 or 3 years for a young girl's periods to settle down after puberty and establish a pattern.

Remedies
• *A daily standard infusion of St John's wort can help relaxation and ease pain during menstruation.*
• *Take 20 ml of black haw bark tincture when period cramps start, repeat if necessary after 4 hours.*

FOOD FADS

Adolescents are especially prone to eating disorders, special diets, or meat aversion, and in all cases nutritional balance may become upset. Caution: Professional help for eating disorders is vital.

Remedies
• *Vegetarian teenagers should eat pulses and grains at each meal. Vegans should take 50 μg of vitamin B[12].*
• *To stimulate the appetite, take 2–5 drops of tincture of a bitter herb such as barberry, in a little warm water before meals.*
• *If tension is adding to the food problem, drink a standard infusion of a relaxing nervine, such as chamomile.*

YOUNG WORKING PEOPLE

THE FOURTH LIFE STAGE

LIFE IS BUSY for people in their 20s and 30s and good health is often taken for granted. Minor ailments are usually shrugged off fairly easily, while more serious conditions are frequently ignored. Maintaining a healthy lifestyle can be difficult when you rush or miss meals, have little time to relax and unwind, consume an excess of alcohol and smoke cigarettes. But neglect and over-

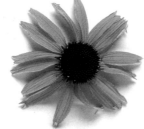

Echinacea flower

indulgence at this stage can lead to long-term problems, as ignored sprains and strains sow the seeds of arthritis, for example, while persistent gastritis can develop into ulcers. Herbs can be used to treat the common, self-limiting problems of healthy adults and they are also useful as gentle tonics – soothing stress and providing energy to help the system cope with peaks of activity.

Preventative Treatments

A healthy diet is essential, but some of the following may help in times of stress. See p. 126 for herbs to avoid in pregnancy.
For dosage advice on remedies, vitamins and minerals, see p. 83. For instructions on making remedies, see pp. 62–79.

HERBS

ECHINACEA boosts the immune system. At the first hint of a cold or flu or if suffering from stress, take 3 x 200 mg capsules 3 times a day.

MILK THISTLE SEEDS are a good restorative for the liver, especially if alcohol intake is high. Take 5 ml of tincture before heading for the party – and again first thing next morning (and don't drink to excess).

CLEAVERS cleanse the lymphatic system. Take 5–10 ml of tincture or pulp a bucketful in a food processor to make a thick green drink. Take 3 times daily.

VITAMINS & MINERALS

B VITAMINS are often deficient if the diet is poor, if alcohol consumption is high or if long-term medication is being taken (including oral contraceptives). Take 400–800 mg vitamin B complex daily.

VITAMIN C helps those prone to infections. Eat plenty of fruit or take 500–1,000 mg daily. Heavy smokers can benefit from higher doses (up to 3 g per day).

ZINC absorption can be affected by high alcohol intake, low protein consumption or dieting. Eat plenty of nuts, pulses and wholemeal bread, or take up to 50 mg daily.

TIMELY TONICS

ASTRAGALUS ROOT
This is an effective energy tonic, popular in China with young adults. Take 1–2 x 200 mg capsules or a sherry glass of tonic wine daily.

Tonic wine

HE SHOU WU
The Chinese believe this helps to increase reproductive energy. Take a sherry glass of tonic wine daily.

Tonic wine

SCHIZANDRA FRUIT
An aphrodisiac for both men and women, this herb also improves ability to cope with stress. Take 2 x 200 mg capsules or a sherry glass of tonic wine daily.

Dried fruit

SIBERIAN GINSENG
An excellent remedy to increase stamina and help the system cope with stress. Take 3 x 200 mg capsules or tablets daily.

Tablets

Health Profile

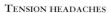
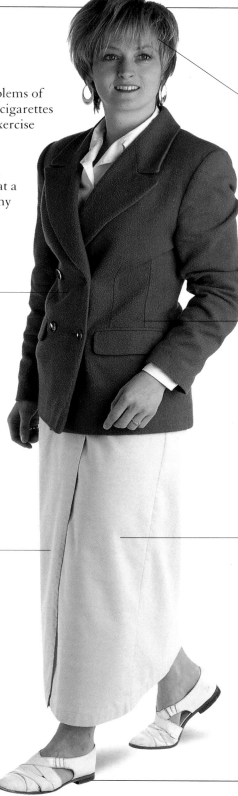

LIVING LIFE to the full can bring problems of excess. Too much alcohol, junk food, cigarettes or caffeine combined with too little exercise or relaxation may soon lead to minor health problems such as gastritis and tension headaches, which if neglected will only get worse. It is essential to eat a balanced diet and try to adopt a healthy lifestyle during this life stage as an investment for later years.

GASTRITIS

Too much alcohol and contaminated food – often inadequately reheated in a microwave – are common causes of acute gastritis, characterized by vomiting and diarrhoea lasting for 1–2 days.

Remedies
• *A cup of cold Indian tea without milk or sugar can help reduce gut inflammation and ease symptoms.*
• *Take 2–3 slippery elm capsules every 3–4 hours or mix a teaspoon of slippery elm powder in a cup of hot water and drink every 3–4 hours while symptoms persist.*

SPRAINED JOINTS AND MUSCLES

Sports and exercise, such as squash, football, tennis and jogging can cause joint injuries, which if not remedied in youth can all too easily lead to arthritis in old age.

Remedies
• *Use elastic tubular bandages to support sprained ankles.*
• *For sprains and strains, mix 5 drops each of rosemary, thyme, sage and lavender oils with 10 ml sweet almond oil and rub in twice a day.*
• *Use arnica cream on bruises and sprains and take a homeopathic Arnica 6x tablet every 4 hours after painful accidents.*

TENSION HEADACHES

Long working hours, deadlines, a stressful journey home and too much caffeine can all cause tension headaches. Learning to relax is an essential part of treatment.

Remedies
• *Mix 5 drops of lavender oil in 5 ml of sweet almond oil and massage the temples and neck.*
• *Drink a cup of chamomile and wood betony infusion for relaxation. (Note: Avoid wood betony in pregnancy.)*

ULCERATIVE COLITIS

Excessive and recurrent diarrhoea and depression are the hallmarks of this debilitating condition that is most common among young adults. It is often stress-related and can be worse in pregnancy.

Remedies
• *Drink a cup of chamomile and agrimony infusion 3–6 times daily.*
• *Take 2–3 capsules of slippery elm 3 times a day or chew a small piece of liquorice stick once or twice a day to ease inflammation.*

PRE-MENSTRUAL SYNDROME

Too much coffee or chocolate, and an irregular or worrying sex life can contribute to pre-menstrual tension, which is often severe in young, childless women. Avoiding artificial stimulants and taking exercise can help.

Remedies
• *Take a cup of* Dang Gui *(Chinese angelica) decoction daily.*
• *Try 10–20 drops of chaste-tree tincture in water each morning.*
• *Take 500 mg of evening primrose oil daily.*
• *Vitamin B[6] can be helpful in some cases. Take 2–10 mg daily, preferably in a B-complex mix.*

PARENTHOOD

THE FOURTH LIFE STAGE

WHETHER FROM preference or financial necessity, young parents frequently combine full-time jobs with the demands of small children, often with very little outside help. In the past, grandparents were usually on hand to help with childcare, but today they may live miles away and be fully occupied with their own lives. For many people, the arrival of children, with the inevitable

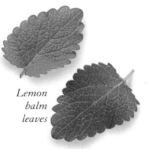

Lemon balm leaves

pressure on time and finances, marks a decline in their social life, and can lead to a growing dissatisfaction with the ties of a young family. Personal interests may become neglected, and it is very important for parents to schedule special "private time" alone together. Herbs can help encourage relaxation for the parents, thereby reducing tension within the family.

Preventative Treatments

No-one who is young and fit should take too many supplements, but a few of these may be useful. See p. 126 for herbs to avoid during pregnancy. For dosage advice on remedies, vitamins and minerals, see p. 83. For instructions on making remedies, see pp. 62–79.

HERBS

LEMON BALM soothes the digestion, and is a good antidepressant, helpful for post-natal problems. Drink a cup of standard infusion daily.

LINDEN FLOWERS calm stressed nerves and reduce the risk of atherosclerosis (hardening of the arteries). Take a cup of standard infusion 2–3 times daily, flavoured with a little peppermint.

EVENING PRIMROSE OIL contains essential fatty acids and can ease menstrual irregularities. Take 250–500 mg daily, for several months.

VITAMINS & MINERALS

VITAMIN E can help to lower raised cholesterol levels – especially in young adults. Take 300–600 IUs daily.

MAGNESIUM levels are sometimes low in PMT sufferers, particularly if the diet is poor. Take 400–800 mg daily.

IRON intake of vegetarians and menstruating women is often insufficient. Eat plenty of wholemeal bread, pulses, egg yolk, parsley, watercress and (if not vegetarian) shellfish, liver and kidney. Alternatively, take up to 40 mg daily.

TIMELY TONICS

DANG GUI
A tonic for the female reproductive system and helpful for anaemia. Take tablets (follow the dosage instructions on the pack). Do not use during pregnancy.

Tablets

MARJORAM OIL
Use 2–3 drops in baths to counter stress or tiredness, or add 5 drops to 5 ml of sweet almond oil and use as a massage oil. (Do not use during pregnancy.)

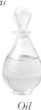

Oil

ROYAL JELLY
A traditional tonic also now believed to improve female fertility. It provides many vitamins and amino acids. Take 1–2 x 250 mg capsules or a 10 ml phial daily.

Capsules

GAN CAO
An excellent energy tonic and detoxifier. Chew small pieces of root or take a sherry glass of tonic wine daily. (Do not take if suffering from high blood pressure.)

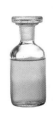

Tonic wine

Health Profile

"Don't panic" should be the motto of every young family, as financial crises loom and toddlers wreak havoc or succumb to endless infections. Regular relaxation is important for both parents, as a build-up of stress can all too often pave the way for nervous disorders and long-term physical problems.

IRRITABILITY

Children can be hard work and test the patience of a saint. Learn to ignore minor irritations and find time for a little personal pampering.

Remedies
• *Drink an infusion of wood betony regularly instead of tea or coffee. (Avoid in pregnancy.)*
• *Add 2–3 drops of lavender or geranium oils to bathwater to soothe frayed nerves.*
• *Try Bach Flower Remedies – beech to reduce intolerance and impatiens for general irritability. Add red chestnut for unnecessary worry or elm for inability to cope.*

LOSS OF LIBIDO

Exhaustion frequently take its toll on a couple's sex life, and it is important to spend time relaxing together.

Remedies
• *Burn a few drops of jasmine and sandalwood oils in a diffuser attached to an electric lamp.*
• *Drink a cup of schizandra decoction 2–3 times a day for a week using 25 g berries to 500 ml water.*
• *Damiana is a good aphrodisiac for men (take 1 ml of tincture in warm water 2–3 times daily); while chaste-tree berries work well on women (take 10 drops of tincture in warm water 3 times a day).*

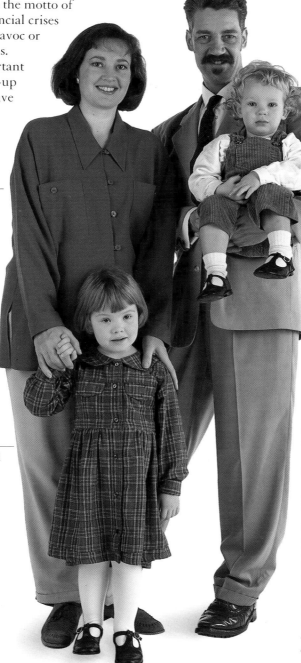

EXHAUSTION

Long working hours, pregnancy and a demanding family can exhaust even the fittest.

Remedies
• *Rest and relaxation are essential. Instead of caffeine, take Siberian ginseng capsules (2 x 200 mg up to 3 times daily) as a boost.*
• *Drink a tea made from equal amounts of dried vervain, rosemary and gotu kola 2–3 times a day. (Note: this quantity of vervain is safe in pregnancy, but do not exceed the dose or take for more than 2–3 weeks.)*

INDIGESTION

Stress and rushed mealtimes soon lead to indigestion with pain, wind and heartburn. In pregnancy, the growing foetus often plays havoc with the digestion.

Remedies
• *Drink a cup of standard fennel or chamomile infusion after meals.*
• *To relieve heartburn and acidity, take 1–2 capsules filled with equal amounts of powdered slippery elm bark and marshmallow root.*
• *Chew crystallized ginger or drink peppermint infusion to relieve wind.*

PEPTIC ULCERS

This painful condition, caused by erratic meals and stress, is most common among people aged 30–40. Ulcers require professional treatment, but the following remedies can relieve symptoms in controlled conditions.

Remedies
• *Make an infusion of 15 g each of dried meadowsweet and chamomile and take a cup up to 4 times daily.*
• *Take 1–2 capsules of 1 g slippery elm and 1 g San Qi 3 times daily.*

THE MIDDLE YEARS - MEN

THE FIFTH LIFE STAGE

SOME MEN experience an emotional crisis mid-life, as they see youth slipping away. This may result in a yearning for days gone by, or even lead to divorce and a search for a new, younger partner. Other men become depressed as they dwell on unfulfilled ambitions and the frustrations of failing strength. Fortunately for many men, the middle years are a very

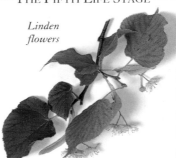

Linden flowers

positive time, encompassing wide interests and achievements, a comfortable lifestyle, and a happy family life, as children become less demanding and dependent. Such self-satisfaction brings its own problems, notably a tendency to take insufficient exercise and to eat too much. Energy-giving herbs can provide a boost, while others relieve the aches and pains of middle age.

Preventative Treatments

Taking care to lead a healthy life is very important. Some of the following may also help guard against illness.
For dosage advice on remedies, vitamins and minerals, see p. 83. For instructions on making remedies, see pp. 62–79.

HERBS

LINDEN FLOWERS are ideal for over-stressed executives, encouraging relaxation and helping to reduce the risk of atherosclerosis. Drink a cup of standard infusion regularly, flavoured with peppermint if required.

OATS are an excellent antidepressant and can also help reduce cholesterol levels. Eat porridge for breakfast or take 5 ml of oat tincture daily.

GARLIC reduces cholesterol levels and is strongly antibacterial, helping combat infections. Use plenty in cooking or take 2–3 garlic pearls daily.

VITAMINS & MINERALS

BETA-CAROTENE (a vitamin A-like compound) is thought to be a valuable cancer preventative. Eat plenty of carrots or take up to 10,000 IUs daily. Caution: Excessive vitamin A can be toxic.

VITAMIN E is helpful in combating coronary artery disease and poor circulation. Take 400 IUs daily. Caution: Avoid, except under medical supervision, if taking blood-thinning drugs such as warfarin.

SELENIUM has been shown to help prevent cancer and reduce the risk of heart attacks. Take 100 µg daily.

TIMELY TONICS

DAMIANA
This is a stimulating, strengthening tonic which is reputedly an aphrodisiac. Take 1–2 cups of standard infusion daily.

Dried herb

KOREAN GINSENG
Korean, or Chinese, ginseng is a Yang tonic. Take 1–2 x 250 mg tablets or capsules a day. Avoid prolonged use if suffering from high blood pressure.

Capsules

GOU QI ZI
These berries are associated with longevity and are a good liver and kidney tonic. Chew 2–3 or take a 200 mg capsule of the powdered herb daily.

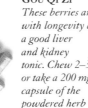

Berries

BENZOIN
A good sedative, especially useful for urinary and respiratory problems. Add 5 drops to the bathwater or use in massage oils.

Oil

Health Profile

TOO MANY BUSINESS LUNCHES and no exercise can result in middle-age spread. The middle years are also a time of severe illnesses, such as heart attacks, lung cancer and digestive problems. Regular exercise and a healthy diet can help to keep these problems at bay.

HIGH BLOOD PRESSURE

Stress and weight gain increase the risk of high blood pressure and heart attacks. It is essential to seek professional help, but exercise, giving up smoking, relaxation and careful weight control are all generally advised. The following remedies can help mild cases.

Remedies
• *Take a standard infusion daily made with equal parts dried hawthorn flowers, linden flowers,* Ju Hua *and yarrow.*
• *Take 2.5 ml each of guelder rose and hawthorn berry tinctures 3 times a day.*

RHEUMATIC ACHES AND PAINS

The middle years are a time when some people are afflicted with rheumatic twinges. They are sometimes associated with developing arthritic disorders and prompt treatment at this stage can prevent problems arising later on.

Remedies
• *Mix 2 ml rosemary oil, 1 ml lavender oil and 2 ml thyme oil in 50 ml sweet almond oil. Massage gently into aching limbs.*
• *Take 2 x 200 mg devil's claw capsules 3 times a day.*
• *Mix 20 ml each of meadowsweet, celery seed, black cohosh, angelica root and bogbean tinctures and take 5 ml 3 times a day.*

EYESTRAIN

In the middle years, the eyes become more long-sighted, and many people need spectacles. It is important to have an eye-test regularly to check that glasses are the right strength.

Remedies
• *Add 5 drops of self-heal tincture to an eyebath of warm water and bathe sore eyes.*
• *Apply used, cold chamomile teabags to the eyes, lie down and relax for 10 minutes.*
• *Drink a cup of* Ju Hua *standard infusion daily.*

PROSTATE PROBLEMS

Benign enlargement of the prostate gland is commonplace, leading to problems with urination. Seeking professional advice without delay is important, to eliminate the possibility of prostate cancer.

Remedies
• *Take 5 ml saw palmetto tincture in a little warm water 3 times a day, or take the herb in the form of over-the-counter tablets (follow the dosage instructions on the pack).*
• *Drink a standard infusion of equal parts of dried damiana and white deadnettle 2–3 times daily.*

CIRCULATORY DISORDERS

Problems with circulation are often associated with smoking, and can manifest as cramp-like pains in the legs. Feet and hands can often be cold, with an increased risk of chilblains.

Remedies
• *Try very hard to give up smoking.*
• *Circulatory stimulants such as prickly ash bark and cinnamon twigs can help: take 2 ml of either tincture 3 times daily in warm water.*
• *Drink a standard infusion of equal parts of dried linden and hawthorn 2–3 times a day.*

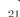

THE MIDDLE YEARS – WOMEN
THE FIFTH LIFE STAGE

FASHION DESIGNER, Coco Chanel, once said that women are born aged 18, 35 or 55. For some women, the middle years start early and they seem to adopt middle-aged attitudes in their teens. Others, however, retain their youthful exuberance to the end. The Chinese traditionally measured a woman's life in seven-year stretches, with the menopause at 49 years

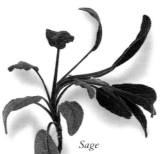
Sage

marking an end to useful and reproductive life. Today, no woman need regard the change of life in such negative terms. Glamorous role models in their middle 50s are commonplace, and although the departure of grown-up children can be traumatic and depressing for some mothers, the middle years are a time of freedom to discover new interests and activities.

Preventative Treatments

It is important to eat a balanced diet. In addition, the following supplements may be useful. For dosage advice on remedies, vitamins and minerals, see p. 83. For instructions on making remedies, see pp. 62–79.

HERBS

SAGE, reputed to guarantee a long life, is also now known to mimic female hormones, making it a useful supplement during the menopause. Drink a cup of standard infusion 1–2 times daily.

ST JOHN'S WORT is restorative and antidepressant, ideal for fraught nerves and menopausal traumas. Take a cup of standard infusion daily.

VERVAIN is a calming nervine and liver tonic and some believe it has a spiritual action. Drink 1–2 cups of standard infusion daily.

VITAMINS & MINERALS

CALCIUM can help reduce the risk of osteoporosis in later life. Green vegetables, nuts and pulses are good sources, or take a 1 g supplement daily.

MAGNESIUM is important for the metabolism of calcium. Leafy green vegetables are important dietary sources. Alternatively, take 400–800 mg daily.

VITAMIN E is an antioxidant and can be useful for reducing menopausal symptoms. Take 400 IUs daily. Caution: Avoid, except under medical supervision, if taking blood-thinning drugs such as warfarin.

TIMELY TONICS

DANG SHEN
The Chinese regard this as a good Yin tonic and a more gentle energy source than ginseng. Take a sherry glass of tonic wine or 2 x 200 mg capsules daily.

Tonic wine

NU ZHEN ZI
A liver and kidney tonic that is also traditionally taken to restore hair colour. Take a sherry glass of tonic wine or 2 x 200 mg capsules daily.

Tonic wine

CHASTE-TREE BERRIES
These stimulate female hormones and can help regulate their production. Take 2 x 200 mg tablets or 2.5 ml tincture in warm water each day.

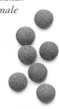
Tablets

CYPRESS OIL
The sedating and calming effect of this oil can help with menopausal problems. Use in massage oils or add 5 drops to the bathwater.

Oil

Health Profile

For some, the middle years can be a time of menopausal problems and emotional upsets, with depression and loss of libido. But they can also be marked by new feelings of independence and self-confidence. A positive attitude to the change of life is essential. Regular exercise is important to maintain bone structure and guard against osteoporosis.

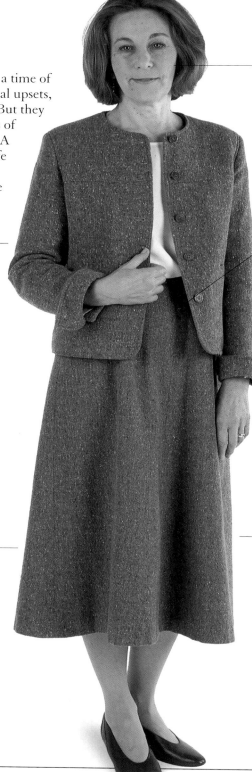

MENOPAUSAL SYNDROME
Menopausal women may experience hot flushes, night sweats, irregular or heavy periods, mood swings and irritability. In traditional Chinese medicine these are linked with a reduction of kidney energy and are treated with tonic, restorative herbs.

Remedies
- *Night sweats can be reduced with sage and mugwort tea. Each evening, drink a large cup of standard infusion made with equal amounts of both herbs.*
- *Chaste-tree berries can help regulate erratic hormones. Take 2.5 ml tincture in a little warm water each morning.*
- He Shou Wu *is a good tonic. Try a sherry glass daily of tonic wine.*

DRYNESS
Dry eyes and a dry vagina are common menopausal problems.

Remedies
- *To help dry eyes, drink a cup of a standard infusion made with equal amounts of dried vervain, wood betony and* Ju Hua *flowers.*
- *Vaginal dryness can be eased by using vitamin E or pot marigold creams. Apply a little morning and evening and before intercourse.*
- *Add 10–20 drops of chamomile oil or 500 ml infusion to bathwater. The infusion may also be used as a vaginal wash.*

ACNE ROSACEA
Starting with a persistent facial flush and progressing to acne-like pustules, this is particularly common during the menopause. Alcohol, tea and coffee make it worse and should be avoided.

Remedies
- *Use a lotion made with 50 ml pot marigold tincture, 50 ml rosewater and 2 drops of rose oil. Apply to the rash 2–3 times a day.*

GALL BLADDER PROBLEMS
"Fat, forty, female and fertile" – the medical student's mnemonic for pinpointing those prone to gall bladder disease says it all. The symptoms include acute colicky pain and professional medical attention is required. Mild conditions may respond to simple home remedies.

Remedies
- *Take 2 ml each of fringe tree bark, fumitory and vervain tinctures in warm water 3 times a day.*
- *To relieve symptoms, drink a cup every 2–3 hours of a standard decoction made from 15 g dried dandelion root, 10 g wild yam root and 5 g barberry bark.*

DEPRESSION
The middle years can feel empty when children leave the nest and partners seem preoccupied with careers. Maintaining a strong image of self-worth is essential.

Remedies
- *Take 2 ml of vervain and oat tinctures with 1 ml of lemon balm tincture, in warm water 3 times daily.*
- *Drink a large cup 3–4 times daily of a standard infusion of equal parts St John's wort and wood betony.*
- *Bach Flower Remedies can help. Try walnut to cope with change, and honeysuckle to stop the mind dwelling on the past.*

THE NEWLY RETIRED
— THE SIXTH LIFE STAGE —

TODAY, RETIREMENT signals a new beginning, a chance to travel to exotic places or develop new interests and hobbies. Retirement, however, is not always trouble-free: it is a time of major re-adjustment, which workaholics in particular often find difficult. Giving up the status and companionship that work brings, or coping

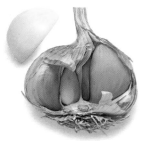
Garlic bulb

on a reduced income, may lead to depression and lack of self-esteem in some people. Maintaining a positive attitude to life is essential. Recent research has associated both prostate problems and osteoporosis with a sedentary lifestyle, so gentle, enjoyable exercise, such as walking, bowls, golf, gardening and cycling is important for both sexes.

Preventative Treatments

A healthy diet is perhaps one of the best investments for a healthy old age. In addition, the following can be useful.
For dosage advice on remedies, vitamins and minerals, see p. 83. For instructions on making remedies, see pp. 62–79.

— HERBS —

GARLIC is especially valuable to help maintain health as old age approaches. Use plenty in cooking or take 2–3 pearls daily.

CINNAMON reduces blood sugar levels and is a useful tonic if the circulation is poor. Try taking powdered cinnamon sprinkled on hot buttered toast.

MOTHERWORT is a tonic herb for the heart and a gentle sedative. It also has a restorative effect on the female reproductive organs. Take a cup of standard infusion regularly.

— VITAMINS & MINERALS —

VITAMIN C, found in fresh fruit and vegetables, is important for everyone, but rheumatism sufferers in particular may benefit from taking a high dose (4 g daily) as it flushes out uric acid from the system and helps with gouty arthritis.

SELENIUM is an antioxidant, preventing cell damage. It is also thought to help maintain a healthy heart and muscles. Take 100–200 µg daily.

VITAMIN B[1] (thiamin) deficiency is linked to heart problems. Take 50 mg daily.

TIMELY TONICS

LING ZHI
Regarded by the Taoists as a tonic for long life, this is ideal at times of change to help resolve the will. Take 2 x 200 mg capsules or 10 ml tincture daily.

Tincture

KOREAN GINSENG
The ideal tonic for the older person. Take 1–2 x 250 mg tablets or capsules or 10 ml tincture daily. Avoid prolonged use if suffering from high blood pressure.

Tincture

BASIL
In India this herb is regarded as a potent spiritual tonic, encouraging faith, compassion and clarity. Take 5 ml of juice daily.

Juice

DANG SHEN
An energy tonic that can be particularly helpful for women and also eases stomach tension. Take a sherry glass of tonic wine or 2 x 200 mg capsules daily.

Capsules

Health Profile

As the body ages, the frustration of aching limbs, lack of stamina, insomnia or failing eyesight can be daunting. Accepting that physical energies are gradually slowing down, staying as healthy as possible and making the most of every day are important lessons. This life stage is a time when any physical abuse will come home to roost: decades of poor diet can lead to late-onset diabetes, for example, and habitual use of laxatives may result in diverticulitis.

ANGINA PECTORIS

Angina, related to disease of the coronary arteries, is characterized by sharp pains in the chest, arms, shoulders or neck. Professional treatment is essential but can be augmented with medicinal herbs.

Remedies
• *If high cholesterol levels are a contributory factor, take 4 x 200 mg garlic capsules or 2 cloves daily.*
• *Drink a standard infusion of equal parts of dried hawthorn, motherwort and linden flowers 3 times a day.*
• *Take 10 drops of San Qi tincture in water 3 times a day.*

LUMBAGO AND SCIATICA

Sciatic pain may run from lower back to knee and is often exacerbated by excessive gardening. Lumbago is a term for pain in the lower back.

Remedies
Add 5 drops each of pine, geranium and peppermint oils to an evening bath and enjoy a long soak. Mix the same oils in 10 ml of infused St John's wort oil and gently massage the affected areas.

ARTHRITIS

Osteoarthritis is caused by general wear-and-tear on the joints and can very quickly limit activity as joints stiffen and pain becomes a misery.

Remedies
• *Take 2 x 200 mg capsules of devil's claw 3 times a day for at least 4 weeks.*
• *Massage infused comfrey oil or comfrey cream into the affected joint twice a day. Continue for at least 2 months.*

LATE-ONSET DIABETES

A tendency to develop this condition can be hereditary. It can also be caused by obesity, and a lifetime of high sugar consumption. Symptoms include excessive thirst, fatigue and increased urination. Professional help is vital.

Remedies
• *Take 2 x 200 mg capsules of fenugreek 3 times a day before meals.*
• *Drink a cup of standard infusion of equal parts dried goat's rue and bilberry leaves 3 times a day.*
• *Eat plenty of garlic, or take 2–3 pearls daily.*

DIVERTICULITIS

Laxatives and a low fibre diet can weaken the lower bowel wall, and small pouches (diverticuli) arise, which become inflamed and infected by trapped food particles.

Remedies
• *Drink a cup of standard decoction of dried wild yam and marshmallow root flavoured with a little liquorice extract 3 times daily.*
• *Drink a cup of standard chamomile infusion regularly to help reduce inflammation.*

THE ELDERLY

THE SEVENTH LIFE STAGE

A CENTURY AGO, most people in the West thought those over 50 were elderly. Today, the number of over-70s in our society continues to grow steadily and many more people live to 80 or 90 years of age. But no matter how vigorous the individual is, the ills of old-age catch up eventually. Despite the skills of modern medicine, cancer and cardiovascular disease

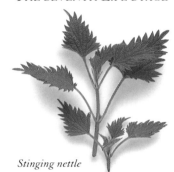

Stinging nettle

remain the developed world's greatest scourges and the risk of suffering from either inevitably increases with age. A varied diet with plenty of fresh fruit and vegetables is now recognized as a preventative factor for both diseases. Unfortunately, apathy often leads to missed meals, so this is a life stage when vitamin and mineral supplements are particularly valuable.

Preventative Treatments

Taking care to follow a healthy lifestyle is very important and the following herbs, vitamins and minerals can further boost health.
For dosage advice on remedies, minerals and vitamins, see p. 83. For instructions on making remedies, see pp. 62–79.

HERBS

STINGING NETTLES are rich in minerals and vitamins and can supplement a deficient diet. Drink a cup of standard infusion daily.

GOTU KOLA is a good nerve tonic used in Ayurvedic medicine to encourage mental calm and clarity. Drink a cup of standard infusion regularly.

KELP, OR BLADDERWRACK is rich in iodine and other minerals and is a gentle metabolic stimulant. It is very helpful in debility. Take 3–6 x 400 mg tablets daily.

VITAMINS & MINERALS

B VITAMINS deficiency can lead to cracking at the corners of the mouth and a sore, red tongue. Take 1–2 tablets of a good quality B-complex supplement.

VITAMIN C is important to combat infection and many progressive diseases. Eat plenty of fresh fruit and vegetables or take 1–2 g supplement daily.

COD LIVER OIL reduces the risk of heart disease. Use combined fish and evening primrose oil capsules (take 500–750 mg daily).

TIMELY TONICS

AMERICAN GINSENG
This has a more Yin character than Korean ginseng and can be preferable for the very elderly. Take 1–2 x 250 mg tablets daily or a sherry glass of tonic wine.

Tonic wine

OATS
Oats are an excellent tonic food, antidepressant and restorative. Make porridge from freshly milled oatmeal and eat regularly.

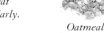

Oatmeal

SAGE
This herb is traditionally associated in the West with longevity. Drink a cup of standard infusion every day.

Dried herb

GINKGO
This herb is known to encourage the circulation of blood to the brain and reduces confusion in the elderly. Take 3 x 200 mg tablets or 10 ml tincture daily.

Tablets

Health Profile

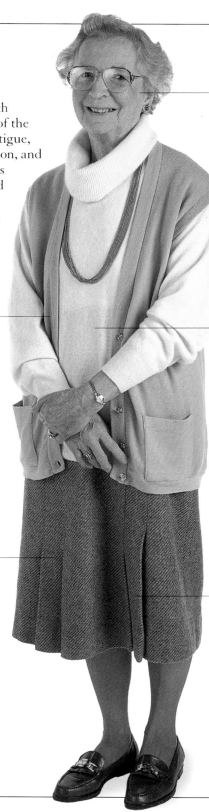

OLD AGE BRINGS its fair share of health problems as energies wane and parts of the body show signs of wear-and-tear. Fatigue, insomnia and poor appetite are common, and general weakness can lead to problems with the digestion, urinary system and circulation. It is important to keep warm and stay as active as possible, and it is also wise to maintain contacts with people of all ages and retain a lively interest in current events.

CONFUSION AND FORGETFULNESS

With age, short-term memory can become impaired. Senile dementia is common and needs understanding and patience from the family as well as professional medical support.

Remedies

• Drink a standard infusion daily of dried ginkgo leaves and wood betony to improve circulation to the brain.
• Add 5 drops each of rosemary and basil oils to bathwater as gentle mental stimulants.

INCONTINENCE

Stress incontinence is common in women who have had children and it affects both sexes in old age. The following herbal remedies can be useful.

Remedies

• Dilute 10 drops of cypress oil in 5 ml of sweet almond oil. Massage into the lower abdomen 2–3 times a day.
• Take 10 ml of horsetail juice twice a day.
• Take a standard decoction of equal amounts of Huang Qi, Dang Gui and Chi Shao Yao 3 times a day to alleviate symptoms.

HEARING PROBLEMS

Deafness and tinnitus limit normal conversation and add to isolation. White noise cassette tapes can ease severe tinnitus and herbs can prove surprisingly helpful.

Remedies

• Combine 25 ml each of tinctures of ginkgo leaves, pasque flower, Nu Zhen Zi, and schizandra berries and take 50 drops in water 3 times daily.
• Take a 200 mg capsule of goldenseal 3 times a day if catarrh is a contributory problem.

CONSTIPATION

Constipation in the elderly can often be caused by general weakness of the digestive system as well as poor diet. Eat plenty of fibre but avoid too much bran, which can be an irritant.

Remedies

• The Chinese used Huo Ma Ren (cannabis seeds) for constipation in the elderly. Sterile seeds are sold by specialist suppliers: make a decoction and drink a cup 3 times a day.
• Take 2.5 ml of Dang Gui tincture in half a glass of warm water 3 times a day.

BRITTLE BONES

Hip fractures are a hazard and severe osteoporosis can lead to a curved spine. Regular exercise and plenty of calcium and magnesium are good preventative measures.

Remedies

• Sage contains oestrogen-like substances that may help prevent loss of calcium from bones. Take a cup of standard infusion daily.
• Take a dessertspoon of freshly crushed linseed daily.

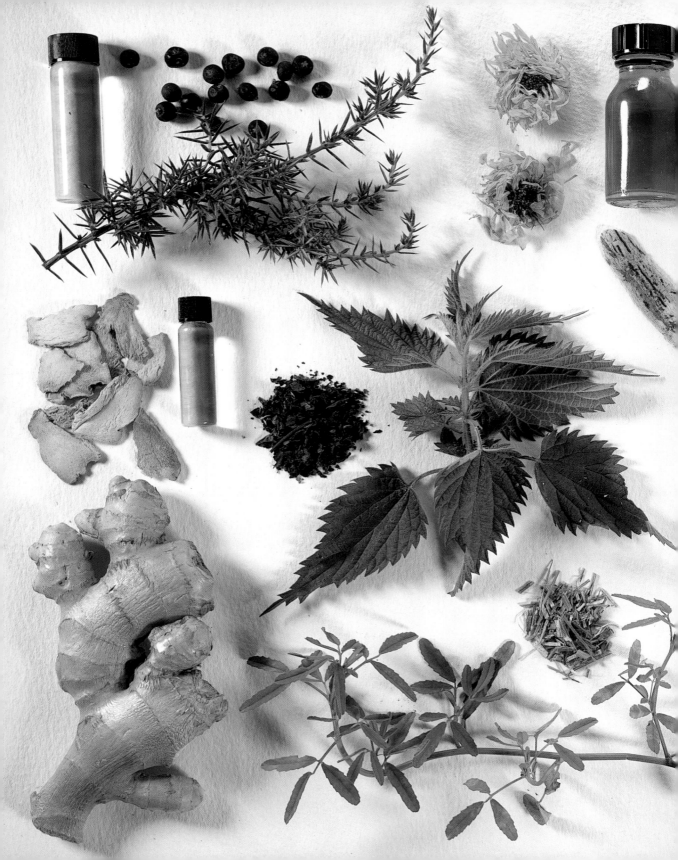

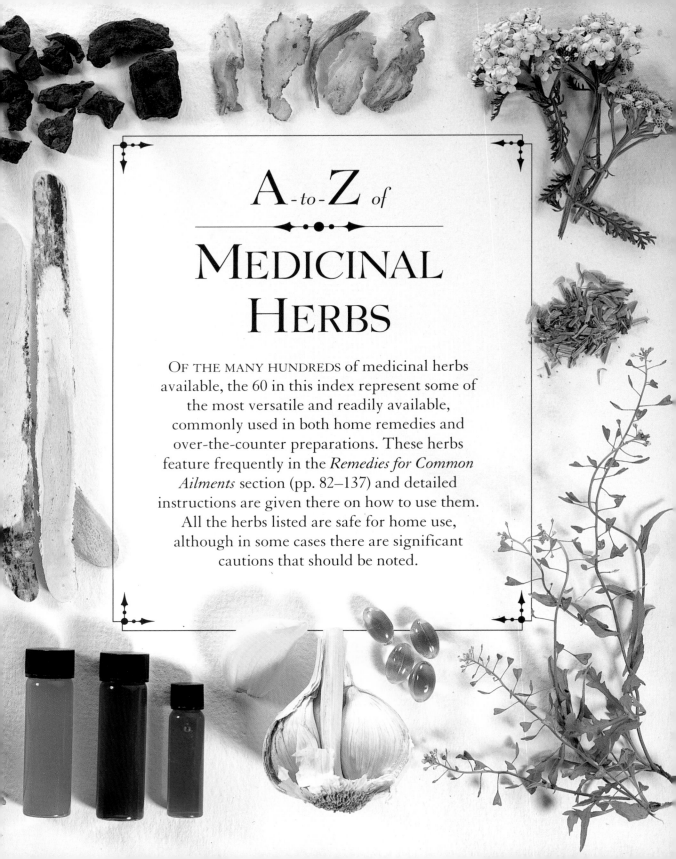

A -to- Z of
MEDICINAL
HERBS

OF THE MANY HUNDREDS of medicinal herbs
available, the 60 in this index represent some of
the most versatile and readily available,
commonly used in both home remedies and
over-the-counter preparations. These herbs
feature frequently in the *Remedies for Common
Ailments* section (pp. 82–137) and detailed
instructions are given there on how to use them.
All the herbs listed are safe for home use,
although in some cases there are significant
cautions that should be noted.

Achillea millefolium
YARROW

Yarrow was once known as "nosebleed", its feathery leaves making an ideal astringent swab to encourage clotting. It is an important herb for treating wounds, taking its name from the Greek hero, Achilles, who used it for just that. The plant was also important in fortune-telling, and yarrow stalks are still used by the Chinese for casting *I Ching* predictions.

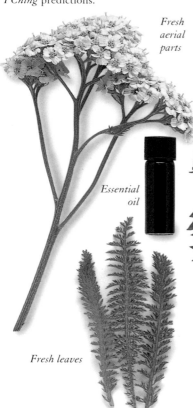

Fresh aerial parts

Essential oil

Fresh leaves

PARTS USED: Aerial parts, essential oil.

KEY USES: Although useful as a wound herb, yarrow is now mostly used for fevers and to relax blood vessels in high blood pressure. It is a bitter-tasting digestive tonic, and is added to remedies to relieve menstrual and urinary disorders.

CAUTIONS:
• Can cause skin rashes.
• Avoid large doses in pregnancy.

Agrimonia eupatoria
AGRIMONY

Agrimony is found growing in hedgerows, its tall yellow summer flowers giving it the folk name "church steeples". It is a member of the rose family and, like all its relatives, is highly astringent. Indeed, it is a valuable wound herb, and was once a much-used remedy on medieval battlefields.

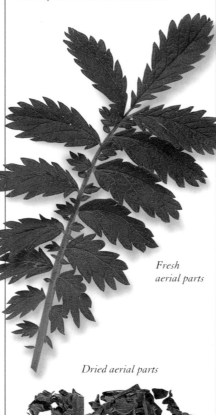

Fresh aerial parts

Dried aerial parts

PARTS USED: Aerial parts.

KEY USES: Like many astringent herbs, agrimony can be helpful for diarrhoea, and it is especially suitable for children. It can effectively stop bleeding from cuts and grazes and, taken internally, can ease heavy menstrual bleeding and acute, severe cystitis.

Allium sativum
GARLIC

The Ancient Egyptians spoke of garlic as a potent remedy for coughs and colds – for which it is still prized today. In many countries garlic is the most popular over-the-counter herbal remedy. Its potent chemicals can only be excreted through the lungs and skin, hence the aromatic consequences of high doses.

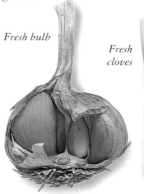

Fresh bulb

Fresh cloves

PARTS USED: Cloves.

KEY USES: Garlic is a good respiratory antiseptic for chest infections and a useful antifungal in candidiasis. It also helps reduce blood cholesterol levels and can be helpful for patients at risk from heart attacks.

Althaea officinalis
MARSHMALLOW

The Romans looked on marshmallow as a culinary delight and the sweet, juicy roots are said to be quite palatable if fried with onions and butter. Medicinally, its mucilaginous (soft, slippery) nature makes marshmallow ideal for soothing respiratory and digestive disorders. It is a very pretty plant – well worth growing in a damp corner of the garden.

PARTS USED: Leaves, root, flowers.

KEY USES: Marshmallow is used as an expectorant for chesty coughs and bronchitis. It is also very soothing for inflamed mucous membranes, especially in the digestive tract and urinary system.

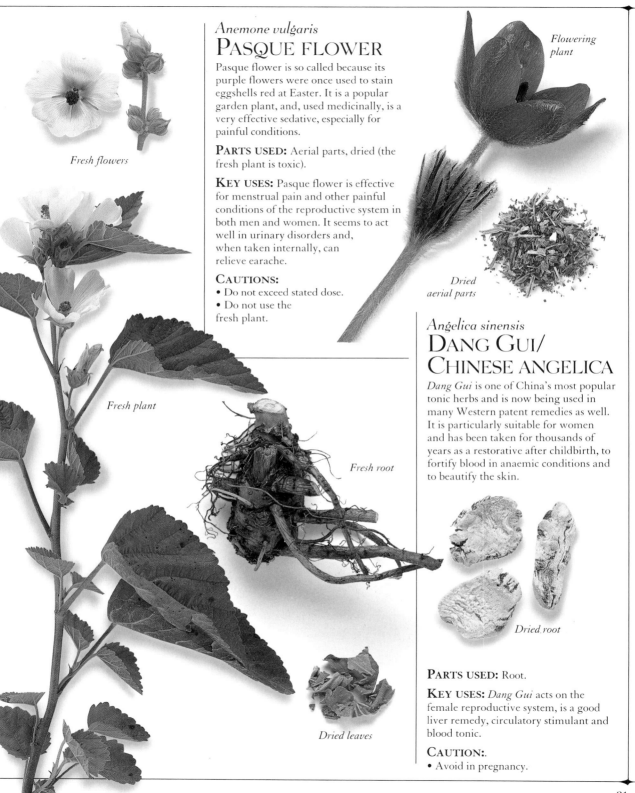

Fresh flowers

Anemone vulgaris
PASQUE FLOWER

Pasque flower is so called because its purple flowers were once used to stain eggshells red at Easter. It is a popular garden plant, and, used medicinally, is a very effective sedative, especially for painful conditions.

PARTS USED: Aerial parts, dried (the fresh plant is toxic).

KEY USES: Pasque flower is effective for menstrual pain and other painful conditions of the reproductive system in both men and women. It seems to act well in urinary disorders and, when taken internally, can relieve earache.

CAUTIONS:
• Do not exceed stated dose.
• Do not use the fresh plant.

Flowering plant

Dried aerial parts

Angelica sinensis
DANG GUI/ CHINESE ANGELICA

Dang Gui is one of China's most popular tonic herbs and is now being used in many Western patent remedies as well. It is particularly suitable for women and has been taken for thousands of years as a restorative after childbirth, to fortify blood in anaemic conditions and to beautify the skin.

Fresh plant

Fresh root

Dried root

Dried leaves

PARTS USED: Root.

KEY USES: *Dang Gui* acts on the female reproductive system, is a good liver remedy, circulatory stimulant and blood tonic.

CAUTION:.
• Avoid in pregnancy.

Apium graveolens
CELERY

Thanks to modern agriculture, celery has now become an all-year-round vegetable. At one time, however, it was only ready for cutting in winter and spring, when it was used as an effective cleansing herbal tonic at a time when little fresh food was available. The seeds are used medicinally. They are harvested after the plant flowers in its second year.

PARTS USED: Seeds.

KEY USES: Celery seed is a diuretic, and is the best remedy for clearing uric acid from the system. It is ideal for gout, arthritis and rheumatism and it can also be useful to treat cystitis and related problems.

CAUTIONS:
• Only use seeds sold for medicinal purposes, as those intended for planting are often treated with fungicide.
• Avoid high doses in pregnancy.

Fresh stalk

Dried seeds

Arnica montana
ARNICA

Arnica is a daisy-like plant, found in rich, peaty, alpine pastures. Taken internally it can be extremely toxic, so it is only used in homeopathic preparations, which are very dilute. In the form of creams and ointments, however, it is one of the most useful in the herbal repertoire.

Fresh flowers

Fresh plant

PARTS USED: Flowers.

KEY USES: Arnica cream can be used for conditions where poor circulation is a contributory factor, such as chilblains, or where the circulatory system needs some stimulation to encourage healing. Arnica cream and an internal arnica homeopathic remedy are a good combination for traumatic accidents.

CAUTIONS:
• Do not use the cream on broken skin.
• Take only homeopathic doses internally.

Arctium lappa
BURDOCK

Burdock and dandelion cordial can still be found in shops occasionally. It is a reminder of what was once a popular spring-cleaning combination, designed to combat constipation and stagnation disorders. The burdock plant is a biennial, growing up to 2 m in height, with a very deep tap root and small pinkish flowers. It is covered in stiff bracts that cling to clothes.

PARTS USED: Leaves, root, seeds.

KEY USES: Burdock is a good cleansing herb for arthritis and various skin conditions; and it is also a digestive stimulant and mild laxative. The root is mostly used although the leaves have a similar, gentler action. The Chinese use the seeds for feverish colds.

Dried leaves

Dried seeds

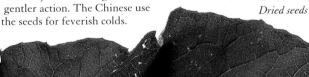

Fresh plant

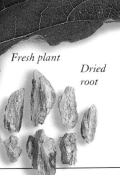

Dried root

Astragalus membranaceus
HUANG QI/ ASTRAGALUS

Huang Qi has been used as an energy tonic by the Chinese for thousands of years, although more recent interest in the herb focuses on its immune-stimulating properties. The plant, known in English as "milk vetch", is a member of the bean family, and can be grown in temperate areas.

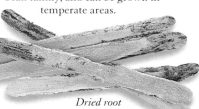

Dried root

PARTS USED: Root.

KEY USES: The Chinese look on *Huang Qi* as a young person's tonic. It is ideal whenever immune-deficiency plays a part in the condition, such as when repeated colds or allergies wear down natural resistance.

Barosma betulina
BUCHU

This tall, South African shrub has a characteristic blackcurrant flavour, making it one of the more palatable medicinal herbs. It originates from Cape Province and was originally used by local Hottentot tribes, both medicinally and in body perfumes.

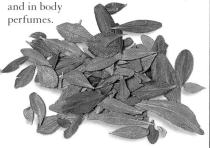

PARTS USED: Leaves.

Dried leaves

KEY USES: Buchu is an effective urinary antiseptic, ideal for cystitis and similar conditions. It is a warming and stimulating herb and makes a useful kidney tonic.

Calendula officinalis
POT MARIGOLD

Back in the 17th century, pot marigold was regarded as an ideal cure for "plague and pestilence", a rather more effective remedy, perhaps, than other plague potions since marigold is highly antiseptic. Its bright orange flowers were also supposed to strengthen the heart, while simply looking at these cheerful plants was recommended to lift the spirits.

PARTS USED: Petals.

KEY USES: Marigold, commonly available as a cream, makes a useful antiseptic, antifungal and astringent remedy for many skin problems, inflammations and minor injuries. Taken internally, it is an effective bile stimulant, useful for the digestive system, and it can also ease menstrual problems.

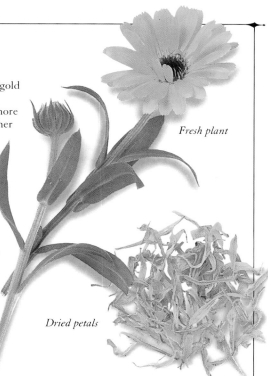

Fresh plant

Dried petals

Capsella bursa-pastoris
SHEPHERD'S PURSE

This common, garden weed has been used medicinally worldwide for at least 2,000 years. In the 17th century, sprigs of it, bound to the hands and feet, were recommended for jaundice, while ointments made from the herb were used on wounds. It is also known as "mother's hearts" because of the shape of its seed pods.

PARTS USED: Aerial parts.

Dried aerial parts

KEY USES: A useful herb to stop external and internal bleeding, shepherd's purse is used mainly to treat urinary and menstrual disorders. It is also a circulatory stimulant and is effective as a wound remedy.

CAUTION:
• Avoid in pregnancy, although it can be helpful during labour.

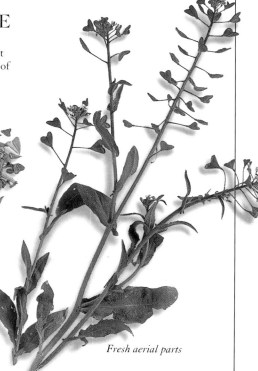

Fresh aerial parts

Capsicum frutescens
CHILLI/CAYENNE

Chilli peppers arrived in Europe from India in the 16th century and were initially used for virulent skin conditions. The herbalist John Gerard disliked the plant, saying that it would "kill dogs". Chillies are, of course, extremely hot and need to be used with caution.

Cimicifuga racemosa
BLACK COHOSH

Black cohosh was used by various Native American tribes for rheumatism, kidney problems, exhaustion and gynaecological disorders. The herb was listed in the US *Pharmacopaeia* from 1820 to 1936. It is a member of the buttercup family, with cream flower spikes and a distinctive black root.

Cinnamomum zeylanicum
CINNAMON

In Roman times, cinnamon was reputed to grow only in remote marshes protected by monstrous bats, a tale that Pliny suggested was circulated by the spice merchants to keep the price high. The bark has been exported from Sri Lanka and India for more than 2,000 years.

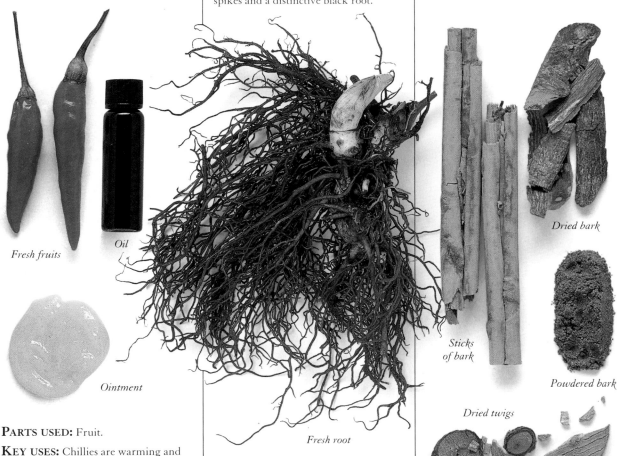

Fresh fruits

Oil

Ointment

Fresh root

Dried bark

Sticks of bark

Powdered bark

Dried twigs

PARTS USED: Fruit.

KEY USES: Chillies are warming and stimulating, and can be taken in remedies for colds, chills, rheumatic pains, poor circulation and nervous shocks. Ointments and oils are used to help stimulate blood flow to an area, or to ease the lingering pain from a shingles attack.

CAUTIONS:
• Avoid touching the eyes or cuts after handling fresh chillies.
• External use may cause dermatitis.

PARTS USED: Root.

KEY USES: Black cohosh is a useful remedy for all sorts of muscle pains and cramps. It is an effective muscle relaxant for spasmodic conditions, including menstrual cramps, and also appears to have some hormonal actions.

CAUTIONS:
• Do not exceed the stated dose.
• Avoid in pregnancy.

PARTS USED: Bark, twigs, essential oil.

KEY USES: Cinnamon bark is a warming digestive remedy. It also has a tonic effect on the kidneys, helps stimulate the circulation, and makes an effective tea for common colds. The diluted essential oil can be used in chest rubs or abdominal massage for colic.

Citrus aurantium
BITTER ORANGE

Bitter oranges are most familiar these days in traditional English marmalade, although the essential oils (neroli distilled from the flowers and bergamot from the fruit) are also well known. The Chinese use both the ripe and immature fruits in medicine.

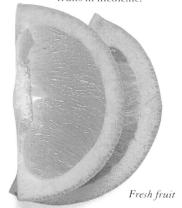

Fresh fruit

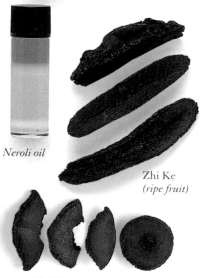

Neroli oil

Zhi Ke (ripe fruit)

Zhi Shi (unripe fruit)

PARTS USED: Fruit, peel, essential oils.

KEY USES: Bitter oranges are carminative for wind and indigestion, and can also relieve nausea. Both neroli and bergamot oils are widely used in aromatherapy, acting on the nervous and digestive systems.

Dioscorea villosa
WILD YAM

The wild yam was the original starting point for making the first oral contraceptives – thanks to the hormonal compound, diosgenin, it contains. The Aztecs regarded it as a relaxing digestive remedy, which is how herbalists still use it today.

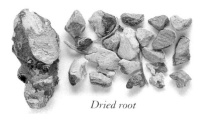

Dried root

PARTS USED: Root.

KEY USES: Wild yam is a good anti-spasmodic for the digestive and reproductive system, especially helpful for irritable bowel syndrome or for menstrual pain.

CAUTION:
• Avoid in pregnancy, although it may be taken during labour.

Eleutherococcus senticosus
SIBERIAN GINSENG

Siberian ginseng is a relative newcomer to the herbal repertoire. Only widely used since the 1930s, it is ideal for combating the stresses of 20th-century life. It was once a favourite with both Soviet athletes and long-distance truck drivers, who took it regularly to increase stamina and improve performance.

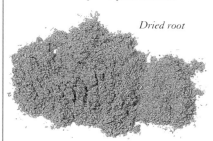

Dried root

PARTS USED: Root.

KEY USES: Ideal whenever stress is proving a problem, Siberian ginseng is a useful herb to take before exams or a busy time at work. It can also be helpful as a remedy for nervous exhaustion and lack of energy.

Echinacea angustifolia
ECHINACEA

The Native Americans used echinacea, also known as "purple coneflower", for snakebites, fevers, and wounds, and the herb soon became popular with the early settlers. Today it is appreciated as an important immune stimulant and antibacterial, ideal for almost any sort of infection.

PARTS USED: Root.

KEY USES: Whenever there is infection – viral, bacterial or fungal – echinacea has a role. It is the ideal choice for colds, 'flu and kidney infections and can be helpful in viral-based arthritis, and for sore throats. It can also be applied externally for some skin conditions.

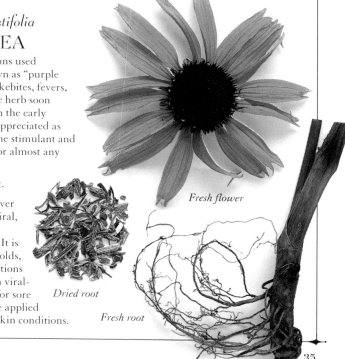

Fresh flower

Dried root

Fresh root

Eschscholzia californica
CALIFORNIAN POPPY

The Californian poppy is a common garden flower. Known as "nightcap" in the USA, it is a gentle and very useful sedative, ideal for sleeplessness, even in children. Unlike some members of the poppy family, it has no addictive side-effects and is quite safe to use.

PARTS USED: Aerial parts.

KEY USES: A gentle sedative for the nervous system, this herb is excellent for insomnia, over-anxiety or tension, and can be pleasantly taken in teas at any time. It can also be very helpful for over-active digestive systems.

Fresh aerial parts

Eucalyptus globulus
EUCALYPTUS

Once a favourite cure-all for the Australian Aborigines, eucalyptus is mainly used today for infections and chest problems. Current research suggests it is a very potent antibacterial. The tree grows well in temperate climates although it is tropical in origin.

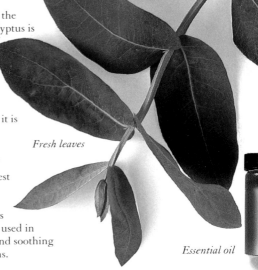

Fresh leaves

PARTS USED: Essential oil.

KEY USES: Eucalyptus is best used as an external remedy. The oil is ideal in chest rubs and inhalants to treat all sorts of respiratory problems and, used in massage oils, it is warming and soothing for rheumatic aches and pains.

Essential oil

Euphrasia officinalis
EYEBRIGHT

Eyebright is a nondescript, semi-parasitic plant found mainly in grass meadows and chalk downland, yet it is one of the most effective anticatarrhals. As its name suggests, it is also used as an eye remedy, and, indeed, was a favourite with great 17th-century herbalists such as Nicholas Culpeper.

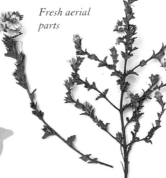

Fresh aerial parts

PARTS USED: Aerial parts.

KEY USES: Eyebright relieves congestion and catarrh and is useful in remedies for hayfever and common colds. It can be taken internally or used in eyebaths as a soothing remedy for many eye infections and irritations.

Filipendula ulmaria
MEADOWSWEET

In the 1830s, anti-inflammatory chemicals were first extracted from meadowsweet, and in the 1890s the world's first patent drug appeared, as "aspirin", taking its name from the old Latin name for meadowsweet, *Spiraea ulmaria*. The herb has always been a favourite for fevers and rheumatic pains, but, unlike modern aspirin, it does not irritate the stomach lining.

PARTS USED: Aerial parts.

KEY USES: A good soothing remedy for the stomach, it is helpful for gastritis, stomach upsets and many other digestive problems. Meadowsweet is also an excellent anti-inflammatory for arthritis and rheumatic conditions.

CAUTION:
• Meadowsweet is rich in salicylates, so avoid in cases of aspirin allergy.

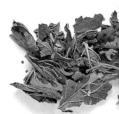

Foeniculum officinalis
FENNEL

The Ancient Greeks called fennel *marathron*, a word believed to mean "to grow thin", and used it as a slimming aid. Medieval churchgoers used to chew the seeds during boring sermons to stop stomach rumbles. Today, Florence fennel is a popular garden vegetable, useful in salads, while the original herb is still important for digestive remedies.

PARTS USED: Seeds.

KEY USES: A useful herb for digestive problems, it is ideal for indigestion, stomach chills, or to relieve griping pains. Fennel is also used to encourage milk flow in nursing mothers and can be taken to help respiratory complaints.

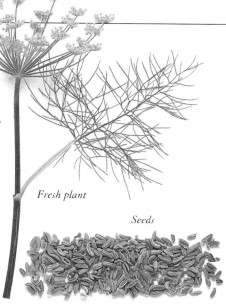
Fresh plant

Seeds

Glycyrrhiza glabra
LIQUORICE

For more than 2,500 years liquorice has been used in medicine, both in Western Europe and in the Far East. The Chinese call it "the grandfather of herbs" and use it in many prescriptions to help balance other ingredients. It is also used to flavour medicines. Liquorice is a member of the bean family and grows well in temperate climates.

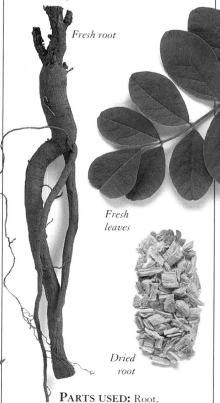
Fresh root

Fresh leaves

Dried root

PARTS USED: Root.

KEY USES: Liquorice is a soothing digestive remedy, helpful for both gastric ulceration and diarrhoea. It is also an expectorant and useful for problem coughs as in bronchitis and asthma. The herb encourages the production of many hormones, such as hydrocortisone, an anti-inflammatory.

CAUTIONS:
• Avoid excessive use in cases of high blood pressure.
• Liquorice should not be taken by people on digoxin-based drugs.

Galium aparine
CLEAVERS

One of the most common weeds, cleavers is also known as "goosegrass" (because geese like to eat it) and "sweetheart" (for the way it clings to shrubs). It has an ancient reputation as a spring tonic, traditionally taken as a cleansing remedy after the long winter.

PARTS USED: Aerial parts.

KEY USES: A good cleansing herb and lymphatic tonic, it is useful in many skin disorders and also for glandular problems, including tonsillitis and glandular fever.

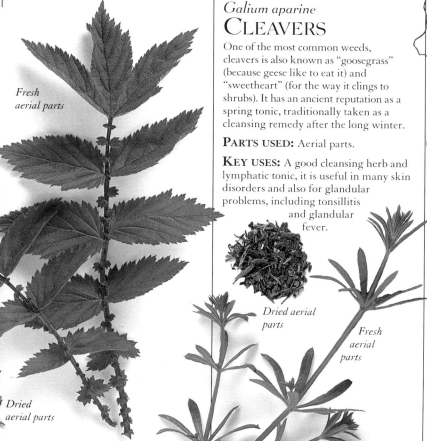
Fresh aerial parts

Dried aerial parts

Dried aerial parts

Fresh aerial parts

Hydrastis canadensis
GOLDENSEAL

One of the most popular digestive remedies among Native American tribes, goldenseal became a favourite with 19th-century herbalists both in America and Europe. The pioneers used to chew it for sore mouths and stomach upsets, although its bitterness would deter most modern sufferers. Goldenseal belongs to the buttercup family and only grows in a warm climate.

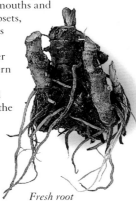

Fresh root

PARTS USED: Root.

KEY USES: A good anticatarrhal and liver stimulant, goldenseal is useful for many respiratory, digestive and menstrual problems, and can also be used externally for some skin conditions.

CAUTION:
• Avoid in pregnancy and in cases of high blood pressure.

Hypericum perforatum
ST JOHN'S WORT

St John's wort was once hung above doorways during midsummer to ward off evil spirits, and the red extract produced from its flowerheads was believed to be ideal for treating wounds and inflammations. Some say its name derives from the Knights of St John of Jerusalem, who used it to heal wounds during the Crusades.

PARTS USED: Aerial parts, flowering tops.

KEY USES: St John's wort is a good external anti-inflammatory, suitable for burns, wounds and joint problems. It is also used for nervous disorders, including depression and anxiety and can be particularly useful for emotional upsets during the menopause. In recent years, extracts have been tested for alleviating immune-deficiency problems.

CAUTION:
• Prolonged use may occasionally lead to photosensitivity.

Hyssopus officinalis
HYSSOP

Hyssop was used as a cure for asthma and catarrh by the Ancient Greeks, although the plant known from the Bible "purge me with hyssop and I shall be clean" (*Psalm* 51) is now believed to be a variety of marjoram. In the past, hyssop was also used for treating some forms of epilepsy. It forms an attractive, shrubby plant, useful in the garden to repel cabbage white butterflies.

PARTS USED: Aerial parts, essential oil.

KEY USES: Hyssop is a valuable respiratory remedy, and is especially good for children. It is a bitter stimulant that can be taken for digestive disorders.

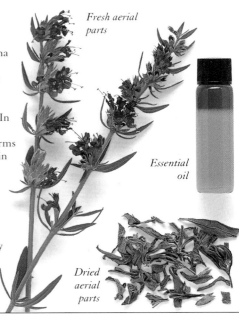

Fresh aerial parts

Essential oil

Dried aerial parts

Fresh aerial parts

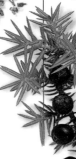

Fresh flower

Dried aerial parts

Juniperus communis
JUNIPER

Juniper has long been associated with ritual purifications and its smoke is still used to purge Eastern temples. It was also used in Ancient Egypt for mummification. Today, the herb is mainly regarded as an important urinary antiseptic, while the essential oil is used for arthritis and psoriasis.

PARTS USED: Berries, essential oil.

KEY USES: The herb is taken internally to alleviate cystitis and urinary infections. Oil from the berries is used for chest problems and aches and pains, while cade oil from the twigs is useful for skin conditions.

CAUTIONS:
• Do not use in pregnancy.
• Avoid using internally for more than six weeks as the herb can irritate the mucous membranes.

Lactuca virosa
WILD LETTUCE

Beatrix Potter's bunnies fell asleep after eating too much lettuce – a good example of this herb's sedative properties! Until the 1930s, extracts of the sap were sold as "lettuce opium", which was recommended as a painkiller and as a treatment for insomnia and anxiety. The herb is most potent as it goes to seed; cultivated lettuce leaves used in salad have little potency.

Fresh aerial parts

PARTS USED: Aerial parts.

KEY USES: Wild lettuce is used as a sedative for anxiety, mania and other nervous problems. It can also be taken to soothe coughs, relax over-active digestive systems, and to relieve muscular pains.

CAUTION:
• Do not exceed the stated dose; overdosage is extremely toxic.

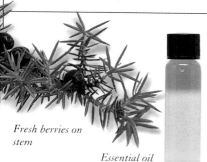
Fresh berries on stem

Essential oil

Lavandula angustifolia
LAVENDER

Lavender is a favourite in herb gardens, where it is prized for its delightful scent. The Romans used it to scent bathwater, hence its name, which comes from the Latin verb to wash (*lavare*). It was prescribed for coughs by the Greeks.

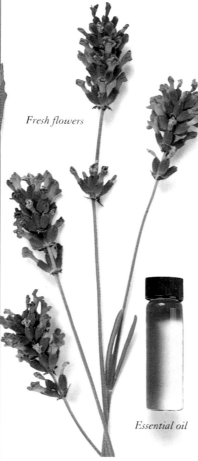
Fresh flowers

Essential oil

PARTS USED: Flowers, essential oil.

KEY USES: Lavender is generally regarded as an effective sedative and calming remedy for the digestion. It is ideal for migraines and headaches, either taken internally or used externally as a massage oil. Lavender oil is also soothing for sunburn, and makes a relaxing and uplifting addition for baths.

CAUTION:
• Avoid high doses in pregnancy.

Lonicera japonica
HONEYSUCKLE

The Chinese have long used honeysuckle flowers (*Jin Yin Hua*) as a cooling remedy for feverish colds, while in the West they have been recommended for chest problems and urinary infections since Roman times. In 17th-century England, Nicholas Culpeper considered "honeysuckle conserve" an essential ingredient for the household dispensary.

PARTS USED: Flowers.

KEY USES: Both the traditional European variety (*L. periclymenum*) and the more familiar Chinese plant can be used for chesty colds and coughs. Honeysuckle is also useful for feverish conditions, including the aches and pains of flu and joint inflammations.

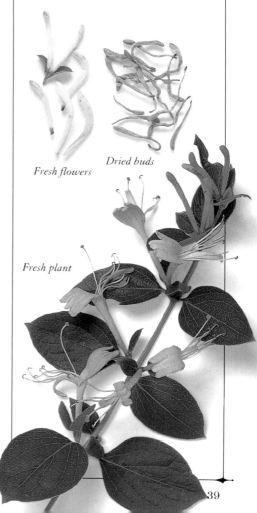
Fresh flowers

Dried buds

Fresh plant

Matricaria recutita
CHAMOMILE

The Anglo-Saxons looked on chamomile, or "maythen", as one of the nine sacred herbs given to heal the world by the god Woden. The plant has a very distinctive smell – described by the Ancient Greeks as "ground apple" – and produces pungent flowers for homemade chamomile tea.

PARTS USED: Flowers, essential oil.

KEY USES: A good sedative and calming herb for the digestive system, chamomile is also a favourite for babies and children, easing colic and teething pains. It is good for insomnia, and is also valuable for skin conditions and irritations.

CAUTIONS:
• Do not use chamomile oil in pregnancy.
• The fresh, growing plant may cause a contact skin rash in sensitive individuals.

Fresh plant

Melaleuca alternifolia
TEA TREE

The healing attributes of oil from the Australian tea tree were first investigated by the French in the 1920s and it has proved to be one of the most popular herbal antiseptics. Today it is widely used in many commercial preparations, and is important as an antifungal and antibacterial in many infectious conditions.

PARTS USED: Essential oil.

KEY USES: It is used as an antiseptic for many skin infections, such as thrush and acne. The oil can also be used in chest rubs or inhalants for colds and makes a useful hair rinse for head lice or nits.

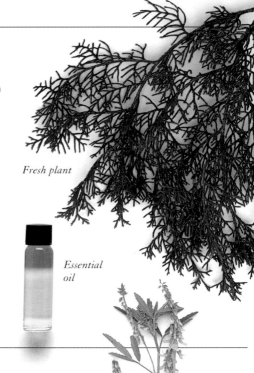

Fresh plant

Essential oil

Melilotus officinalis
MELILOT

Also known as "king's clover", melilot is a striking, yellow field plant, which gives off a characteristic smell of new-mown hay as it dries. It was once the main ingredient of a favourite all-purpose household ointment, and today it is still used for treating skin conditions as well as varicose vein problems.

PARTS USED: Aerial parts.

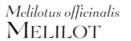
Fresh aerial parts

KEY USES: The herb helps to repair damage to blood vessels so it can be helpful for varicose veins or in creams for varicose eczema. Melilot is also used for some types of menstrual pain, depression and insomnia, and is especially suitable for the elderly.

CAUTION:
• Melilot should not be taken by people on anticlotting drugs such as warfarin.

Dried leaves

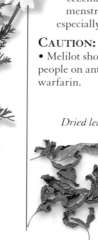

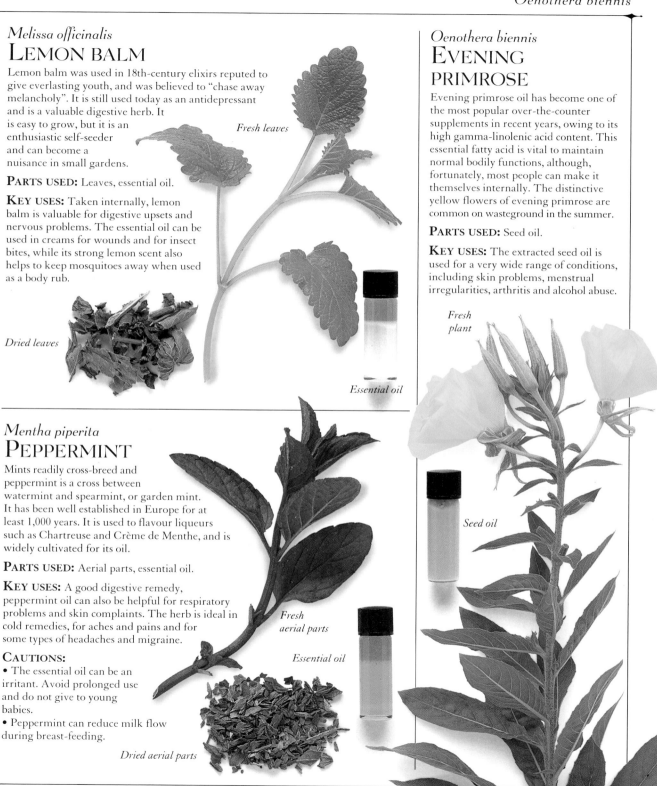

Melissa officinalis
LEMON BALM

Lemon balm was used in 18th-century elixirs reputed to give everlasting youth, and was believed to "chase away melancholy". It is still used today as an antidepressant and is a valuable digestive herb. It is easy to grow, but it is an enthusiastic self-seeder and can become a nuisance in small gardens.

Fresh leaves

PARTS USED: Leaves, essential oil.

KEY USES: Taken internally, lemon balm is valuable for digestive upsets and nervous problems. The essential oil can be used in creams for wounds and for insect bites, while its strong lemon scent also helps to keep mosquitoes away when used as a body rub.

Dried leaves

Essential oil

Oenothera biennis
EVENING PRIMROSE

Evening primrose oil has become one of the most popular over-the-counter supplements in recent years, owing to its high gamma-linolenic acid content. This essential fatty acid is vital to maintain normal bodily functions, although, fortunately, most people can make it themselves internally. The distinctive yellow flowers of evening primrose are common on wasteground in the summer.

PARTS USED: Seed oil.

KEY USES: The extracted seed oil is used for a very wide range of conditions, including skin problems, menstrual irregularities, arthritis and alcohol abuse.

Fresh plant

Seed oil

Mentha piperita
PEPPERMINT

Mints readily cross-breed and peppermint is a cross between watermint and spearmint, or garden mint. It has been well established in Europe for at least 1,000 years. It is used to flavour liqueurs such as Chartreuse and Crème de Menthe, and is widely cultivated for its oil.

PARTS USED: Aerial parts, essential oil.

KEY USES: A good digestive remedy, peppermint oil can also be helpful for respiratory problems and skin complaints. The herb is ideal in cold remedies, for aches and pains and for some types of headaches and migraine.

CAUTIONS:
• The essential oil can be an irritant. Avoid prolonged use and do not give to young babies.
• Peppermint can reduce milk flow during breast-feeding.

Fresh aerial parts

Essential oil

Dried aerial parts

Panax ginseng
GINSENG

Ginseng has been known in the West since the days of Marco Polo, although its widespread use dates only from the 18th century. The Chinese have used the root (*Ren Shen*) of this plant as an energy tonic for at least 5,000 years and today it forms the basis of many patent remedies. Most roots are now commercially cultivated, as wild plants are scarce.

Fresh root

PARTS USED: Root.

KEY USES: This strong energy tonic has been popular with elderly Chinese for centuries. It is also a good lung remedy and can help to speed recovery in chronic chest conditions.

CAUTIONS:
• Avoid high doses or prolonged use in pregnancy.
• If taking ginseng regularly, it is best to take a short break from the herb every couple of months, and limit other herbal stimulants and caffeine.

Petroselinum crispum
PARSLEY

Like nettles, parsley robs the soil of many minerals and vitamins and concentrates them in its leaves, making this traditional garnish a healthy part of a meal. The Ancient Greeks associated the plant with death and glory, and used it as fodder for their warhorses and decoration for their tombs. It does not like being transplanted, so is best sown where it will grow.

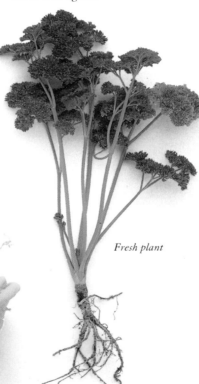

Fresh plant

PARTS USED: Leaves.

KEY USES: A good diuretic and dietary supplement, parsley can be helpful for many urinary problems as well as fluid-retention associated with menstrual irregularities. Its concentrated minerals make it a valuable supplement for anaemia. It also encourages milk flow in nursing mothers.

CAUTION:
• High consumption of the leaf is best avoided in pregnancy.

Plantago spp.
PLANTAIN

Once known as "waybread", common plantain (*P. major*) was one of the Anglo-Saxons' sacred herbs. The Native Americans called it "white man's foot" because it followed the settlers. Both common plantain and the taller ribwort species (*P. lanceolata*) are used medicinally; common plantain is used in first aid to treat bee stings, while ribwort plantain is important as a digestive and respiratory remedy for a range of catarrhal conditions.

Fresh leaf (P. lanceolata)

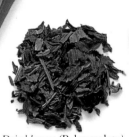

Dried leaves (P. lanceolata)

PARTS USED: Leaves.

KEY USES: Ribwort plantain is a good anticatarrhal for colds and allergic rhinitis. It is also a soothing digestive remedy for various types of gastric irritation and inflammation and makes a useful external poultice for stings and slow-healing wounds.

Polygonum multiflorum
HE SHOU WU/ FO TI

He Shou Wu (known as *Fo Ti* in the USA) is one of the most important Chinese tonic herbs and is believed by the Taoists to bring longevity and wisdom. It was traditionally drunk daily as a tonic wine and was reputed to dispel grey hairs and increase reproductive energy. Its English name is "fleeceflower".

Dried root

PARTS USED: Root.

KEY USES: As a tonic herb, *He Shou Wu* can be especially helpful for menopausal women. It is believed by the Chinese to boost creative energy, so it is useful for hard-working executives suffering from creativity "burn-out". In China it is also given for some heart disorders and used externally for sores.

CAUTION:
• Only the prepared variety, obtainable from Chinese herb shops, should be used.

Fresh leaf
(P. major)

Rosmarinus officinalis
ROSEMARY

Rosemary has long been regarded in Europe as a stimulating herb that helps to dispel melancholy. According to Gerard in the 16th century it "maketh the harte merrie". The herb traditionally signified remembrance, and was exchanged by lovers or left on tombs. Its stimulant properties are due to chemicals in the aromatic oil, which is extracted and used in aromatherapy.

Fresh aerial parts

Essential oil

Dried aerial parts

PARTS USED: Aerial parts, essential oil.

KEY USES: The herb is a good digestive tonic and a carminative. It also helps stimulate the nervous system, and was traditionally believed to improve failing memory. Externally, the essential oil is good for arthritis, rheumatism and some sorts of headache.

Rumex crispus
YELLOW DOCK

A common hedgerow weed, yellow dock takes its name from its root rather than its nondescript flowers. It was traditionally included in spring tonics, which were gentle laxative and nutritive mixes, taken to combat the effects of a poor winter diet. Today it is a useful digestive remedy that is also used as a cleansing herb for a range of toxic conditions.

Root

Fresh plant

PARTS USED: Root.

KEY USES: Yellow dock is mainly used as a cleanser, for skin conditions like eczema and psoriasis, as well as for arthritis and rheumatism. It is a mild laxative and digestive stimulant, useful for constipation and any symptoms of a generally sluggish system.

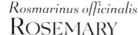
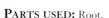
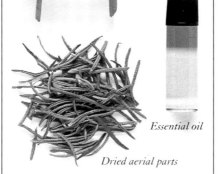

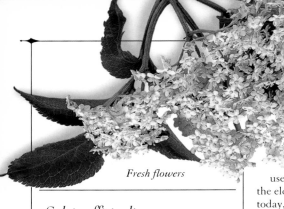

Fresh flowers

Sambucus nigra
ELDER

Once known as "nature's medicine chest" because of the usefulness of its various parts, only the elder's flowers are widely used today, although herbalists sometimes still make traditional "green ointment" from the young stems and leaves. The tree is common in hedgerows, and its rich purple berries are ideal for making winter wine or jam.

PARTS USED: Flowers.

KEY USES: Elderflowers are excellent for all sorts of catarrhal conditions, including colds, flu and hayfever. They help to reduce fevers and inflammations and can be used both internally and externally. The berries make a palatable source of vitamin C in winter.

Scutellaria lateriflora
SKULLCAP

Virginian skullcap arrived in Europe in the 17th century from the USA and was known as "mad dog herb" from its reputation as a remedy for rabies. Today, the herb is used for nervous disorders with the native European species, *S. galericulata*, reputedly having similar properties. The name derives from the scoop-shaped seed pods that resemble skullcaps.

PARTS USED: Aerial parts.

KEY USES: It is an excellent sedative and antispasmodic, ideal for all sorts of nervous tension, anxiety, over-excitability, insomnia and stress-related problems.

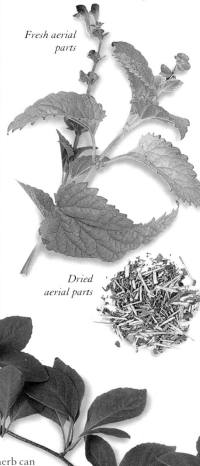

Fresh aerial parts

Dried aerial parts

Salvia officinalis
SAGE

Like other herbs associated with "women's problems", a thriving sage bush in the garden was believed to show that "the mistress was master" and ruled the house. Drinking sage infusions regularly was recommended for a long life and the herb was once regarded as a panacea and general tonic.

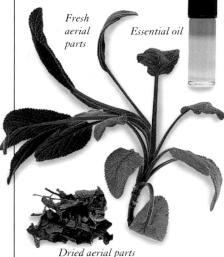

Fresh aerial parts

Essential oil

Dried aerial parts

PARTS USED: Leaves, essential oil.

KEY USES: Sage's actions tend to focus on the mouth, throat and female reproductive system, and it is used to treat symptoms from mouth ulcers to menopausal sweats. Like many culinary herbs it is also a good digestive remedy, stimulating bile flow and regulating its action. Externally, sage is useful as a hair rinse and ointment for insect bites.

CAUTIONS:
• Avoid taking high doses in pregnancy.
• Sage should not be taken by epileptics.

Schisandra chinensis
SCHIZANDRA/WU WEI ZI

One of the most popular tonic herbs in China, schizandra berries are well known as an aphrodisiac and were once also taken regularly by wealthy Chinese women to beautify the skin. The Chinese name, *Wu Wei Zi*, means "five taste fruit", although the predominant flavour is actually quite sour.

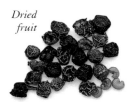

Dried fruit

Fresh plant

PARTS USED: Fruit.

KEY USES: Schizandra is a good all-round relaxing tonic, useful for insomnia and anxiety. It can also live up to its reputation as a sexual invigorator. The herb can be helpful in allergic or irritant skin conditions, and can also be added to cough remedies.

Stachys betonica
WOOD BETONY

One of the most popular medieval herbs, wood betony was at one time recommended for almost everything, from insanity to prostate problems. It was often worn as an amulet to ward off disease and was recommended in the *Grete Herbal* of 1516 for "those that are fearful". Uncommon in herb gardens today, it is a very pretty plant, with bright pink flowers in midsummer.

PARTS USED: Aerial parts.

KEY USES: Today, wood betony is mostly used as a sedative and as a digestive remedy. It has a tonic effect on the circulation, especially in the brain, making it useful for headaches and as a tonic for the elderly.

CAUTION:
• Avoid high doses in pregnancy.

Fresh aerial parts

Dried aerial parts

Taraxacum officinale
DANDELION

Dandelion's country name of "piddley bed" testifies to its traditional use as a potent diuretic. It is a relatively recent arrival to the herbal repertoire, known to be used medicinally in Europe only since the 15th century. Although the herb is usually classed as a weed, the young leaves are good to eat in salads.

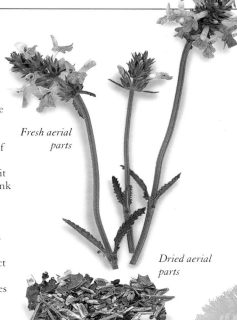

Fresh flower

Fresh root

Fresh leaf

PARTS USED: Leaves, root.

KEY USES: The leaves, which are rich in potassium, are a more potent diuretic than the root. The latter makes an excellent liver tonic, useful for a variety of digestive complaints. The herb is also a good cleanser for skin and arthritic problems.

Tanacetum parthenium
FEVERFEW

Early herbalists, like John Parkinson in the 17th century, believed feverfew was far too bitter to eat raw and recommended frying the leaves first. Today, it is an extremely popular remedy for migraine. It is commonly grown as a garden plant and can be confused with chamomile.

Fresh flowers

Fresh plant

PARTS USED: Leaves.

KEY USES: Taken regularly, feverfew can reduce the risk and severity of migraine attacks. It is also strongly anti-inflammatory and can be helpful in rheumatoid arthritis. The tea can be taken for menstrual pain.

CAUTION:
• Fresh feverfew can occasionally trigger mouth ulcers. Stop taking the herb if this happens. • Feverfew should not be taken by those taking warfarin or similar anti-clotting remedies.

Thymus vulgaris
THYME

Thyme is an excellent antiseptic herb for the respiratory system and for centuries it has been used for treating bronchitis and troublesome coughs. Some scholars argue that the name comes from a Greek word meaning "courage", because the herb is such a stimulating tonic.

PARTS USED: Aerial parts, essential oil.

KEY USES: As well as being an important respiratory remedy, thyme is a good digestive herb, warming and astringent for stomach chills and diarrhoea. The oil is extremely antiseptic and antifungal, and can be applied well diluted to wounds.

CAUTION:
•Avoid high doses in pregnancy.

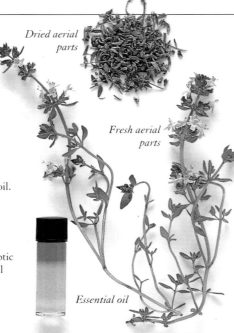

Dried aerial parts

Fresh aerial parts

Essential oil

Urtica dioica
STINGING NETTLE

Gardeners may condemn stinging nettles as "robbing the soil" of nutrients, but their greedy feeding helps concentrate a wealth of minerals and vitamins in the plant, making it an ideal remedy for many deficiency problems. Some nettle varieties were spread through Europe by the Romans who used them as a warming, if painful, body rub in cold climates and until recently, "urtication", or beating with nettles, was a standard folk remedy for arthritis and rheumatism.

PARTS USED: Aerial parts.

KEY USES: A circulatory stimulant and diuretic, stinging nettles are often used for treating irritant skin conditions. They also clear uric acid from the sytem, thereby relieving gout and arthritis. The nutrient-rich leaves make a useful tonic for general use or in anaemia.

Tilia europaea
LINDEN

The linden, or lime, tree is a familiar sight, growing on streets in many European cities, with characteristic winged seeds that appear in autumn. The tea is popular in Europe, where it is often known by its French name *tilleul,* and is drunk as a soothing after-dinner infusion.

PARTS USED: Flowers.

KEY USES: Linden is a useful sedative for nervous tension and anxiety. It helps reduce the build-up of fatty deposits in blood vessels (atherosclerosis) and relaxes the blood vessels, making it a particularly good remedy for high blood pressure associated with stress. The herb is also helpful in fevers.

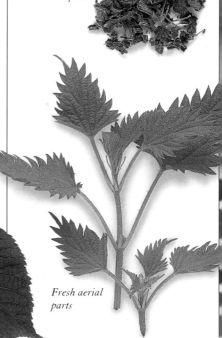

Dried aerial parts

Fresh aerial parts

Fresh plant

Verbena officinalis
VERVAIN

Once sacred to the Druids, vervain was used in fortune-telling and witchcraft well into the 17th century. Traditionally, it was gathered during the "dog days" in July for maximum potency. The original species is a drab, weedy plant, but related ornamental varieties are widely available.

PARTS USED: Aerial parts.

KEY USES: Vervain is a good liver stimulant and a relaxing nerve tonic and is used for a range of digestive problems, as well as depression and tension. It can also be used to ease labour pains, to alleviate various skin conditions, and is regarded as spiritually uplifting.

CAUTION:
• Avoid high doses in pregnancy.

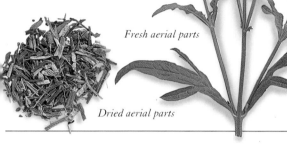

Fresh aerial parts

Dried aerial parts

Viola tricolor
HEARTSEASE

This herb was once a favourite addition to love potions, hence its common name, while the Ancient Greeks used it to reduce anger and soothe headaches. The plant was considered to symbolize pleasant thoughts. It also has a long history as a respiratory remedy.

PARTS USED: Aerial parts.

KEY USES: Heartsease is a useful expectorant for chesty coughs and can be helpful for a wide range of infected or inflamed skin conditions. It is a mild, cleansing diuretic and contains rutin, which is a good restorative for capillary membranes.

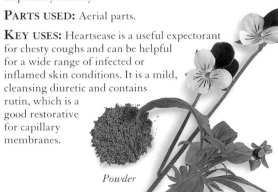

Powder

Fresh aerial parts

Zea mays
CORNSILK

Indian corn, or maize, was once the staple food of many Native American tribes, vital in the diet and also used as a medicine. Ground corn was used by the Aztecs for dysentery and urinary infections, and the early European settlers were quick to recognize its importance.

PARTS USED: Stamens.

KEY USES: The fine, silky stamens are mainly used as a soothing diuretic, for irritant bladder conditions like cystitis, and for prostate problems. They can sometimes be helpful for bedwetting children.

Dried stamens

Zingiber officinalis
GINGER

An important Chinese herb, ginger has been used in the West for more than 2,000 years, both medicinally and in cooking. Traditionally, it was added to many complex remedies to reduce toxicity or side-effects. It is a tropical plant but in cooler climates can be grown in conservatories or greenhouses.

PARTS USED: Root, essential oil.

KEY USES: A very warming herb, ideal for colds and chills or as a circulatory stimulant. It helps reduce nausea, so can be taken for travel or morning sickness. It is also a calming digestive remedy, reducing wind and indigestion.

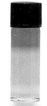

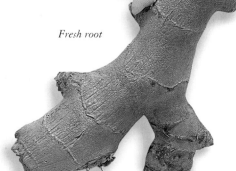

Fresh root

Essential oil

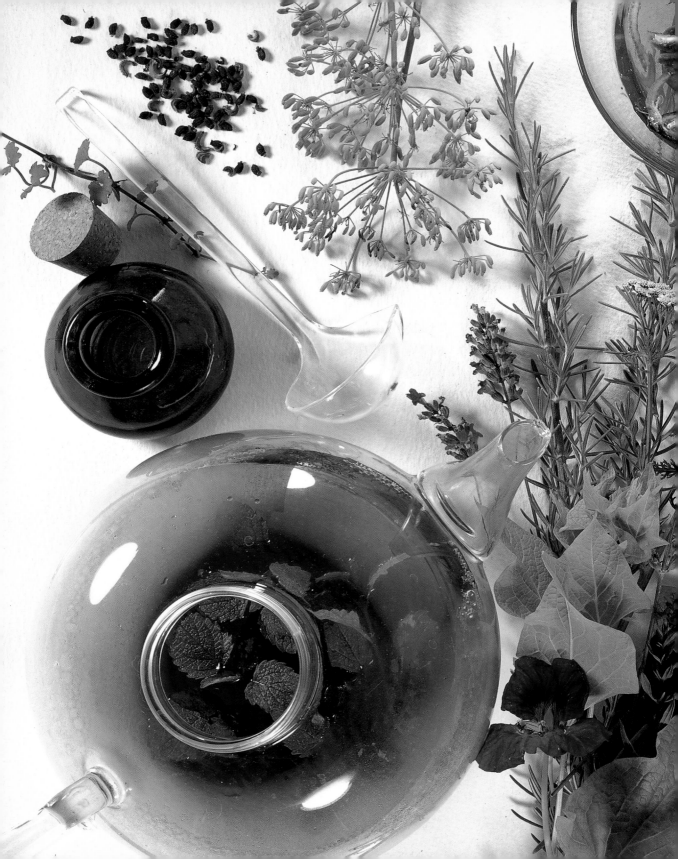

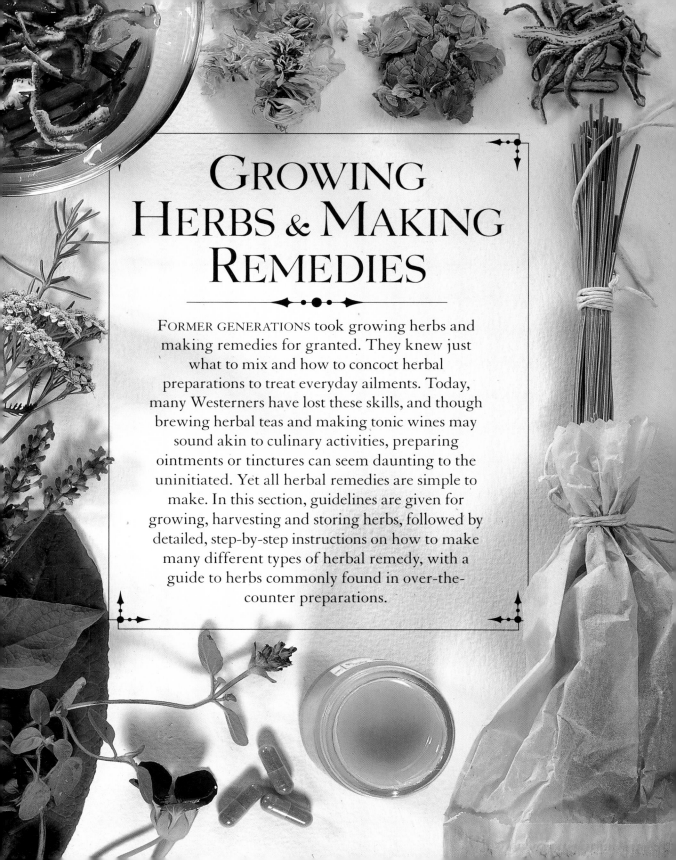

GROWING
HERBS & MAKING
REMEDIES

FORMER GENERATIONS took growing herbs and making remedies for granted. They knew just what to mix and how to concoct herbal preparations to treat everyday ailments. Today, many Westerners have lost these skills, and though brewing herbal teas and making tonic wines may sound akin to culinary activities, preparing ointments or tinctures can seem daunting to the uninitiated. Yet all herbal remedies are simple to make. In this section, guidelines are given for growing, harvesting and storing herbs, followed by detailed, step-by-step instructions on how to make many different types of herbal remedy, with a guide to herbs commonly found in over-the-counter preparations.

GROWING HERBS

THERE IS NOTHING MORE pleasant than being able to snip a few herbs from your own garden or windowbox for a therapeutic tea or a healing ointment. Home-grown and freshly dried herbs have the advantage of being far more potent than commercially grown herbs, which may have been stored for many months before sale, and, for the less common medicinal herbs, home cultivation is often the most practical way to ensure a constant supply of plants. Growing herbs is not difficult and there are many varieties that look very attractive, as well as providing a constant array of delightful and healing aromas to enjoy within the garden.

The medicinal herb garden

Most gardens boast an impressive variety of medicinal plants. There can be hardly any, for example, that do not have shepherd's purse, cleavers, dandelion, stinging nettle or chickweed lurking in some weedy corner – all of which have valuable therapeutic properties. In addition, many of the commonly grown culinary herbs, such as basil, sage, thyme and parsley, may be used medicinally.

Some important therapeutic plants, however, such as chamomile, hyssop and wood betony are unlikely to be found in the garden by chance, and have to be cultivated. It is also worthwhile to consider growing wild flowers in the herb garden, such as agrimony, meadowsweet,

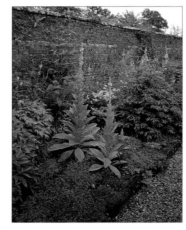

The distinctive yellow spikes of mullein growing in a medicinal herb garden.

melilot and St John's wort, partly for convenience and also because the hedgerows where they grow wild may be polluted.

When planning a herb garden, it is important to take account of the size that chosen plants will grow to, and whether they prefer light or shade. A common misconception is that herbs are drab plants, but it is possible to buy variegated and unusual varieties to add colour and interest. If you are planting medicinal herbs for the first time, try the ten herbs listed, right. Other easily grown plants that are particularly useful include: garlic, heartsease, lady's mantle, marjoram, mullein, peppermint, rosemary, self-heal, vervain and yarrow.

Helpful houseplants

Potted plants have been grown in homes for centuries, but modern research has revealed a new use for them: it has been shown that many plants absorb polluting chemicals from the atmosphere, converting them to harmless substances. Growing plants in town centre offices or inner city homes can therefore help improve the environment for the people who live or work there.

Aloe vera absorbs a wide variety of pollutants from the atmosphere. It is an especially versatile houseplant, useful in first aid for burns (see p. 136). **Spider plants**, **azaleas** and **weeping figs** remove formaldehyde from the atmosphere. This is produced by some building materials, and is also found in some cleaning agents and cigarette smoke. **Common ivy** rapidly clears benzene emitted in some car exhaust fumes. **Peace lily,** or **white flag,** soaks up trichloroethylene from dry cleaning fluid.

Planting a herb garden

The ten useful herbs below will make a good basis for a medicinal herb garden. For general guidelines on growing and harvesting herbs, see pp. 52–7.

Chamomile The flowers can be used to make a delicious and soothing infusion to encourage sleep and ease indigestion.

Fennel A dramatic centrepiece for the garden. Collect the seeds for digestive complaints.

Hyssop An attractive, low-growing shrub. Harvest the aerial parts during summer to use in remedies for chest and digestive ailments.

Lemon balm Use the leaves for a restoring and antidepressant tea. Note: This plant self-seeds prolifically and can get out of hand.

Pot marigold An astringent, healing herb; taken internally for digestive problems or mouth ulcers. It can also be applied externally in creams to treat skin disorders.

Purple sage The leaves are used in mouthwashes. Protect with straw or sacking during harsh winters.

Rosemary Use to make hot infused oils for arthritis. Protect young plants with sacking in winter.

St John's wort Use the fresh flowers to make an infused oil that is invaluable for treating burns and inflammations. Harvest during mid-summer and use the leaves to make a relaxing tea.

Skullcap A sedative for stress and tension. Harvest during flowering when the distinctive skullcap-shaped pods are forming.

Thyme This is one of the best antiseptics in the herbal repertoire. It is useful for lung infections, as a digestive tonic and as a mouthwash.

Medicinal windowbox

Flat-dwellers and those with small gardens may like to plant medicinal herbs in a windowbox. Herbs will grow happily for one or two seasons in containers, but fresh planting each spring is recommended to ensure healthy plants. Herbs thrive in poor soil and a loam-based compost is suitable. If using a peat-based compost, add one part grit to five parts compost to improve soil texture and drainage.

MEDICINAL WINDOWBOX Choose slow-growing varieties of herbs and look out for some of the attractive variegated varieties available. Plant the taller herbs at the back and put trailing plants near the edge.

PEPPERMINT *leaves may be used in teas for indigestion, nausea and headaches.*

LEMON BALM *has a wonderful aroma and tastes good in teas. Choose the variegated variety which retains the plant's medicinal properties but will not grow as vigorously.*

WOOD BETONY *adds colour to the windowbox and the leaves can be collected to make a relaxing tea to counter stress and tension.*

PURPLE SAGE *is a must; it is used in gargles for sore throats, hair rinses and teas. A slow-growing herb, it is suitable for windowboxes.*

THYME *eases coughs and chest complaints and is useful in mouthwashes.*

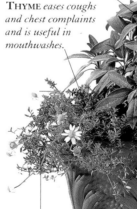

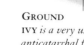

ROMAN CHAMOMILE *is a low-growing perennial that will provide a steady stream of flowers throughout summer for tea-making.*

SELF-HEAL *is an attractive plant, useful in eyebaths for inflamed or tired eyes.*

GROUND IVY *is a very useful anticatarrhal for colds. Use the leaves in infusions or tinctures.*

Buying plants

Although it is always satisfying to grow herbs from seeds or cuttings, some herbs are slow-growing or difficult to propagate, in which case it is well worth buying plants to help establish the herb garden quickly. A visit to a good specialist nursery also reveals a wide range of decorative varieties of herbs: it is worth looking out for variegated lemon balm and mugwort, red ribwort plantain, and the various pink, white and blue-flowered varieties of hyssop, lavender and rosemary, which can all help to add a dash of colour to the herb garden.

■ Look for strong, healthy specimens with plenty of new growth and space in the pot for expansion.

Straggly, yellowing herbs will give disappointing results when planted in the garden.

■ Examine plants for pests: red spider mite, aphids and whitefly tend to congregate on the underside of leaves or on new growth.
■ Check on roots and potting practices by upturning the pot and tapping it gently so that the plant slides out. Healthy root growth should be evident and the compost should hold its shape.
■ Check that plants are correctly labelled. Try to have some idea of what the plant should look like before buying, and if you are unsure ask nursery staff to check.
■ Most specialist herb nurseries expect a peak in sales in mid- to late-spring and will gear production to these times. It is advisable to buy herbs at this time of year, as later in the season plants are likely to become pot-bound. Good nurseries will regularly pot up their products to larger containers as the season progresses, but the price of the herbs usually rises accordingly.

Growing from seed

It is not worth buying annual herbs in pots – as with other annuals they are far better grown from seed. With patience, many perennial herbs may be grown from seed too, although taking cuttings or dividing established plants is sometimes more efficient.

■ Seeds for common medicinal herbs are generally available from garden centres – bear in mind that some, such as melilot and wood betony, will probably be sold in the wild flower section. Specialist herb nurseries can help with hard-to-find seeds.
■ Most annual herbs should be sown in spring, directly where they are intended to grow. Perennials fare better if sown in late summer, potted on and kept in a greenhouse during the winter, before being planted out in the spring.
■ Annual medicinal and salad herbs to sow regularly include: anise, basil, borage, Californian poppy, coriander, corn salad, dill, German chamomile, nasturtium, pot marigold and salad rocket.

■ Although a biennial, parsley is best sown annually – ideally in the place where it is intended to grow. Other biennials to grow from seed include angelica, melilot and mullein.
■ Perennial herbs to grow from seed include: elecampane, fennel, fever-few, hyssop, lady's mantle, sage, St John's wort, self-heal, skullcap and thyme.

SOWING SEEDS

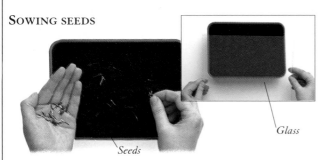

Seeds

Glass

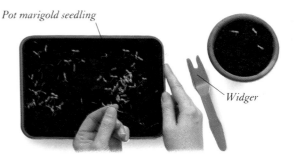

Pot marigold seedling

Widger

1 Fill a seedtray with well-watered compost. Sprinkle on the seeds. Cover large seeds with a fine layer of compost (do not cover small seeds). Cover the tray with glass. Alternatively, place the tray in a plastic bag and store in a warm place (up to 20°C/70°F).

2 Fill a pot with compost. Gently pick up a seedling with a widger, insert it in a small hole in the compost and firm the soil round it.

Pruning & controlling

Some herbs grow rapidly and need vigorous pruning and controlling. In medicinal herb cultivation, regular cropping of plant material to dry for future use, usually limits the need to do too much pruning. In general, cut herbaceous herbs back to 10–15 cm high when collecting aerial parts. Where specific parts of a plant only are used (e.g. lavender flowers), normal gardening rules for pruning apply.

■ Prune rosemary, sage and lavender after flowering in late summer, cutting back to 10–20 cm of new growth.
■ Self-seeders such as fever-few, lady's mantle, lemon balm, mullein and skullcap will colonize the entire garden if not controlled.

■ Some herbs such as mint, and soapwort grow so rapidly that they choke other plants. Confine to small areas of the garden.
■ Avoid pruning rue on damp sunny days as this can cause skin rashes. Clip after flowering.

PRUNING HERBS

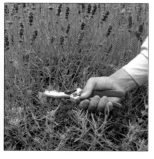

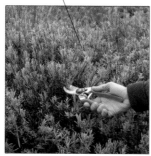

Lavender

1 Using secateurs, cut the dead flower stalks to 10–20 cm of new growth in late summer or early autumn.

2 Early the following spring, cut back shoots by 2.5 cm. Ensure that some green growth remains.

Root division

Many herbs are best propagated by root division. Use a small fork to lever clumps of chives apart in autumn or divide lovage roots with a sharp spade in the early spring when growth has just started. Replant after division and water thoroughly. Other herbs propagated in this way include lemon balm and thyme. To propagate elecampane, Roman chamomile and peppermint, take the runners they develop and replant.

Taking cuttings

Woody perennial herbs are best propagated by cuttings rather than seed. Cuttings can be selected from the side shoots of bushy herbs like sage or rosemary, when semi-ripe in late summer or early autumn, or from the new softwood growth in spring and early summer when growth must develop quickly if the cutting is to survive. Using semi-ripe cuttings is usually more successful for medicinal herbs such as elder, hyssop, lavender, lemon verbena, rosemary, purple sage and thyme.

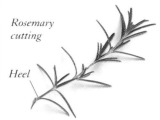

TAKING CUTTINGS

1 Select a suitable shoot. Break or cut it off, keeping a heel of the main stem attached if possible.

Rosemary cutting

Heel

2 Dip the base of the cutting in hormone rooting powder.

Hormone rooting powder

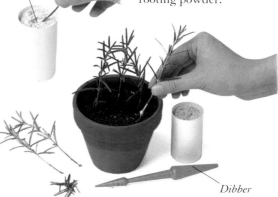

Dibber

3 Fill a 10 cm pot with compost. Make a hole with a dibber and insert a cutting. Insert further cuttings until the pot is filled. Water well. After a few weeks roots should appear at the base of the pot. Pot on the individual cuttings into 75–100 cm pots.

HARVESTING & DRYING HERBS

SEASONAL GROWING PATTERNS mean that it is not possible to use fresh herbs all the year round. Crops have to be harvested, dried and stored for use when fresh plants are unavailable. Herbs should always be dried as quickly as possible, to avoid valuable aromatic chemicals evaporating, and to limit oxidization of important constituents.

The time when herbs are harvested can affect the composition of active chemicals considerably. In many cultures, complex rites accompany the gathering of medicinal herbs, which are, in part, associated with magical traditions, but which also usually ensure that herbs are harvested at their most potent.

Herbs should be collected on a dry day, after the dew has dried, at the peak of maturity when the concentration of active ingredients is at its highest. Dry them quickly away from bright sunlight, allowing plenty of air to circulate. An airing cupboard with the door open is ideal, otherwise a warm room where they will be undisturbed is suitable. A dry garden shed with a low-powered fan running can be used, but it is not advisable to use a garage, as herbs may become contaminated with petrol fumes. Keep the area in which the herbs are dried at 20–32° C/70–90° F.

Most herbs can be dried completely in 5–6 days, although seeds take longer. It is not recommended to dry herbs in a microwave oven. Some researchers have found that this sort of radiation can transform the chemicals in herbs into other substances.

When to harvest

Most herbs are harvested in the summer, either before or during flowering. Seeds and most types of bark are collected in early autumn, and roots in early autumn or spring. The leaves of evergreens such as rosemary, sage and thyme can be collected at any time (but do not gather large amounts when there is a risk of frost).

EARLY SPRING
Roots: dandelion.

LATE SPRING
Aerial parts during flowering: lungwort, sweet violet.
Flowers: coltsfoot, cowslip, elder.

EARLY TO MIDSUMMER
Aerial parts/leaves before flowering: agrimony, angelica, catmint, cleavers, dandelion, dill, fennel, feverfew, garlic, hyssop, lady's mantle, lemon balm, motherwort, parsley, peppermint, plantain, sage, stinging nettles, white horehound, yellow dock.
Bark while flowering: guelder rose.
Flowers/flowering tops: borage, chamomile, honeysuckle, linden, pot marigold, St John's wort.

MID- TO LATE SUMMER
Aerial parts while flowering: Californian poppy, heartsease, marjoram, marshmallow, meadowsweet, melilot, mugwort, shepherd's purse, skullcap, thyme, vervain, wild lettuce, wood betony, wormwood, yarrow.
Flowers: hops, lavender, mullein.
Leaves after flowering: borage, coltsfoot, cowslip, fenugreek, lungwort, sweet violet.

AUTUMN
Roots/bulbs when leaves have wilted: angelica (first year), black cohosh, burdock (first year), comfrey, cowslip, elecampane (2–3 year-old roots), garlic, goldenseal, lovage, marshmallow, purple coneflower, soapwort, tormentil, valerian.
Seeds/fruit when ripe: bitter orange, celery, dill, elder, fennel, fenugreek, hawthorn, lovage.

Flowers

Flowerheads are generally gathered when the plant is in full bloom (see p. 54), and are usually dried whole. Gather them in the morning when they are fully open, after the morning dew has dried. Carefully cut each flowerhead off the stalk, remove any insects or grit and place on a tray lined with absorbent paper. Small flowers, such as lavender, are dried in the same way as seeds – by hanging them upside down and collecting the flowers in a paper bag.

DRYING FLOWERS

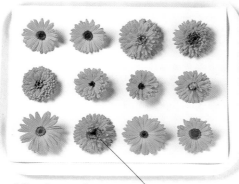

Pot marigold flowers

1 Carefully place each flowerhead on a paper-lined tray – it does not matter if they are touching. Leave to dry in a warm place – an airing cupboard is ideal – and turn regularly.

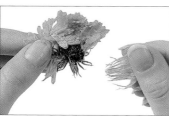

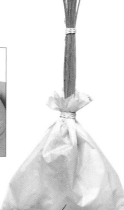

2 When the flowers are completely dry, store in a dark, airtight container. If using pot marigolds, remove the dried petals from the central part of the flower before storing.

Lavender flowers – dry on the stem in a paper bag

Aerial parts & leaves

Gather leaves of deciduous herbs just before flowering and evergreen herbs, such as rosemary, throughout the year (see p. 54). Large leaves, such as burdock, can be harvested and dried individually; smaller leaves, such as lemon balm, are best dried on the stem. If using all the aerial parts, harvest when the plant is flowering, giving a mixture of leaves, stems, flowers and seedheads.

DRYING AERIAL PARTS & LEAVES

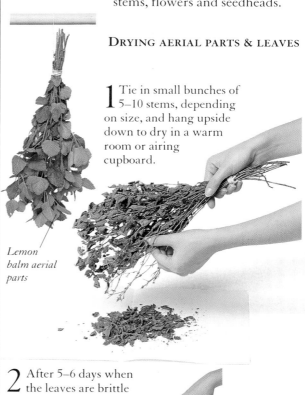

1 Tie in small bunches of 5–10 stems, depending on size, and hang upside down to dry in a warm room or airing cupboard.

Lemon balm aerial parts

2 After 5–6 days when the leaves are brittle to the touch, but not so dry that they turn to powder, rub them from the stem on to paper and discard the larger pieces of stem. If all aerial parts are being used, crumble leaves and stem together.

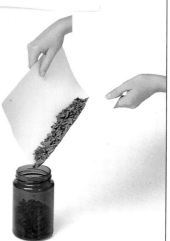

3 Pour or spoon the dried herbs from the paper into a dark, airtight storage container.

Seeds

Seeds are usually harvested in the early autumn (see p. 54). When the seeds are nearly ripe, cut the seedheads with about 15–20 cm stalk, tie them in small bundles with string and hang them upside down over a paper-lined tray. The seeds fall off when they are dry.

DRYING SEEDS

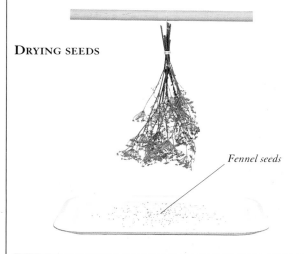

Fennel seeds

Berries

Berries are harvested when they are just ripe, in the early autumn, before they have become too soft to dry effectively. Spread on paper-lined trays, discarding any that show signs of mould. Heat up the oven and then turn it off, placing the trays in the cooling oven with the door ajar for 3–4 hours. Transfer the trays to an airing cupboard or warm room, turning the berries at regular intervals to ensure even drying.

DRYING BERRIES

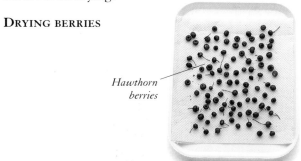

Hawthorn berries

Roots

Except for dandelion roots, which are harvested in spring, roots are gathered in the autumn, when the aerial parts have died down and before the ground becomes hard, making digging difficult. After they have dried completely, some roots reabsorb moisture from the atmosphere, so it is important to check them regularly and discard any that become soft.

DRYING ROOTS

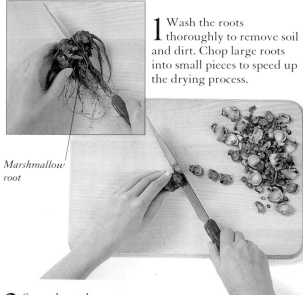

1 Wash the roots thoroughly to remove soil and dirt. Chop large roots into small pieces to speed up the drying process.

Marshmallow root

2 Spread out the root pieces on a paper-lined tray. Heat up the oven and then turn it off. Put the roots into the cooling oven, leaving the door ajar, for 2–3 hours (4–6 hours for larger roots). Transfer to a warm room or airing cupboard until dry.

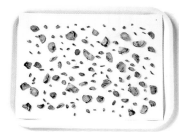

Bulbs

Bulbs should be dug up after flowering when the aerial parts have died down. Collect garlic cloves quickly as they tend to sink downwards once the leaves have wilted and can be difficult to find.

Bark

To avoid damaging the plant or tree, bark should be harvested in the autumn when the sap is falling. Never remove all the bark – or a band of bark completely surrounding a tree. Dust or wipe bark to remove moss or insects, trying not to get it too wet, and then break it up into pieces about 2–5 cm square. Spread the bark pieces on paper-lined trays and leave to dry in an airing cupboard or warm room.

Sap & gel

Sap may be collected from a variety of plants and trees. To collect sap from a tree, make a deep incision with a knife or drill a hole into the bark and then, depending on how much liquid is expected, tie a cup or bucket to the tree to collect the sap. Sap should only be collected in the autumn to minimize damage to the tree. Sap may also be taken from latex plants such as wild lettuce and greater celandine – simply squeeze the plant over a bowl. (It is a good idea to wear protective gloves as some saps are corrosive.) The gel from the *Aloe vera* plant is very useful in first aid (see p. 136) and can also be used to make creams.

COLLECTING GEL

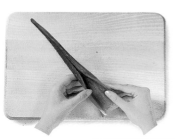

1 Carefully slice along the centre of a leaf and peel back the edges.

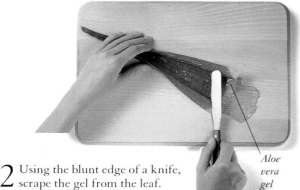

2 Using the blunt edge of a knife, scrape the gel from the leaf.

Aloe vera gel

Freezing herbs

It is possible to freeze small quantities of some medicinal herbs, but the method is more suitable for culinary herbs. Freeze whole sprigs of fennel or parsley and basil leaves in plastic bags.

Buying dried herbs

It is not always possible to grow all the herbs needed for medicinal use – garden space may be limited and some herbs do not thrive in all climates – so buying dried herbs is often necessary.

■ Always buy the minimum quantity you need to avoid lengthy unnecessary storage.
■ Steer clear of shops that sell herbs from clear glass jars in direct sunlight, or shops where the herbs look as if they have been on the shelves for a long time. Herbs tend to lose their colour with age and poor storage, and drab, dusty-looking herbs are a sign that they are well past their prime.
■ Poorly harvested and stored herbs can easily become contaminated: check for mouse droppings, signs of mould, insect infestation or excessive amounts of other plant material – dried grass mixed with eyebright, for example.
■ Try to check that herbs are correctly labelled – mistakes do happen. Some herbs have obvious visual clues (look out for the characteristic seedpods in skullcap and shepherd's purse, for example), and others have distinctive smells. Buy from a reputable shop or specialist mail order supplier, and if possible get some idea of what the herb should look like before buying.

Storing herbs

Herbs should be stored in airtight, dry containers in cool conditions away from direct sunlight. Most will keep for 12 months with little deterioration. Dark glass or ceramic containers are preferable; if using clear glass containers keep them in a dark cupboard away from the light. Inspect herbs regularly for any signs of mould or insect infestation, including eggs and chrysalises – a common problem especially with organically grown or imported herbs. Label dried herbs with details of variety, source and date. Note: For information on how to store herbal preparations (infusions, tinctures, creams, ointments, etc), see pp. 62–79.

HERBAL TEAS

HERBAL INFUSIONS, OFTEN known as herbal teas, are not only taken to treat specific ailments. They also make delicious and healthy alternatives to tea or coffee for regular drinking during the day or after meals. Herbal teas have a wide range of flavours and it is worth experimenting to discover a mix you enjoy. Fresh herbs may be dried at home for teas and ready-made teabags are also available from health food stores and grocers. Most of the commercial blends, though, depend on fruit peel and berries for flavour and can be very rich in sugar – they are best avoided in some conditions, such as candidiasis. For step-by-step instructions on making herbal teas, see p. 64.

Karkade

In the Middle East, travellers are often welcomed with a glass of "karkade", a delicious traditional tea that is cooling and cleansing. It is made from hibiscus flowers.

~ INGREDIENTS ~
50 g dried hibiscus petals
25 g sugar or honey
2 litres water

~ HOW TO MAKE THE TEA ~
Soak the hibiscus petals in 1 litre of cold water for 1–2 hours and then heat to boiling point. Strain and reserve the liquid. Return the petals to the pan adding 1 litre of fresh water and again bring to the boil. Strain and combine the 2 petal extracts adding the sugar or honey. Karkade is traditionally served chilled, but it may also be drunk hot.

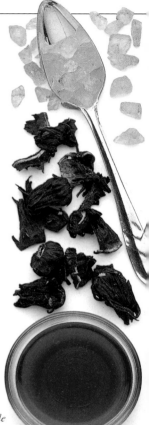
Karkade

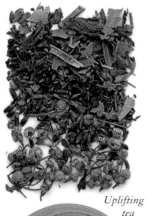
Uplifting tea

Uplifting tea

A restoring brew to improve well-being and happiness, with herbs traditionally believed to lift the spirits.

~ INGREDIENTS ~
25 g dried chamomile flowers
50 g dried vervain
50 g dried peppermint leaves
50 g dried & crushed linden flowers
25 g dried lavender flowers
25 g dried lemon balm leaves
water

~ HOW TO MAKE THE TEA ~
Mix the herbs and store in a dark jar. Place 1–2 teaspoons in a tisane cup or small teapot, add a cup of freshly boiled water and infuse for 5–10 minutes. Strain.

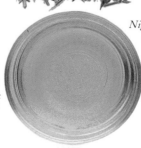
Nightcap tea

Nightcap tea

A hot infusion of relaxing herbs can be just the thing to guarantee a good night's sleep. This mixture is adapted from a recipe of the great French herbalist, Maurice Mességué.

~ INGREDIENTS ~
25 g dried Californian poppies
50 g dried wild lettuce leaves
25 g dried hawthorn flowers
25 g dried melilot
water

~ HOW TO MAKE THE TEA ~
Mix and store the herbs. Place 1–2 teaspoons in a tisane cup or small teapot, add a cup of freshly boiled water and infuse for 5–10 minutes. Strain. Drink hot before going to bed.

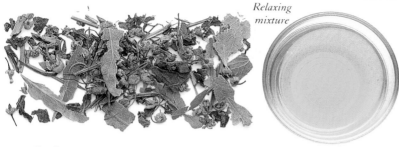

Relaxing mixture

Morning tea

This combination contains stimulating and digestive herbs to provide a refreshing and reviving start to the day.

~ INGREDIENTS ~

25 g dried peppermint leaves
50 g dried hibiscus flowers
50 g dried & crushed strawberry leaves
25 g dried & crushed raspberry leaves
25 g dried marigold petals
25 g dried chamomile flowers
25 g dried cornflowers
water

~ HOW TO MAKE THE TEA ~

Mix and store the herbs in a dark glass or ceramic jar. Place 1–2 teaspoons in a tisane cup or small teapot, add a cup of freshly boiled water and infuse for 5–10 minutes. Strain. Drink first thing in the morning.

Morning tea

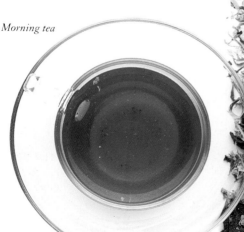

Relaxing mixture

Try this calming mixture of sedating and calming herbs to help unwind after a hard day's work.

~ INGREDIENTS ~

50 g dried lemon balm leaves
50 g dried chamomile flowers
50 g dried & crushed linden flowers
water

~ HOW TO MAKE THE MIXTURE ~

Mix the herbs and store in a dark jar. Place 1–2 teaspoons in a tisane cup or small teapot. Add a cup of freshly boiled water and infuse for 5–10 minutes. Strain.

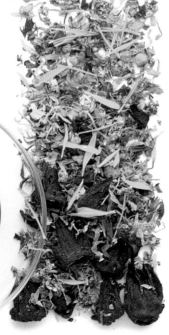

Herbal teabags

Many herbs are available ready-packed in teabags. Although the flavour is generally not as good as using freshly dried or home-grown herbs, they are a convenient option for travelling, or for use at work. The following are often available:

CHAMOMILE – *very relaxing, carminative and soothing. Fresh flowers have a potent and delicious flavour although the dried herb can be disappointing. If the taste is offputting, combine with a little standard Indian tea.*

ELDERFLOWER – *can be an acquired taste; elderflower is effective as an anticatarrhal or for hayfever sufferers.*

FENNEL – *ideal as an after-dinner tea for those prone to indigestion.*

LEMON BALM – *a good uplifting herb to give a refreshing start to the day. It is sometimes combined with fennel in commercial products to soothe digestion.*

LINDEN – *makes a relaxing after-dinner infusion, often combined with peppermint to improve the flavour.*

PASSIONFLOWER – *usually combined with other herbs, such as linden or chamomile, to make an effective night-time brew.*

PEPPERMINT – *a popular herbal tea that can help indigestion and head colds. Do not use to excess (follow the instructions on the pack) as it can be irritant.*

ROSEHIP & HIBISCUS – *a popular commercial combination that is very cooling and refreshing in hot weather.*

VERVAIN – *a good liver stimulant and soothing for the nerves; popular after-dinner – especially in France. Commercial teabags often combine this herb with peppermint.*

WOOD BETONY – *a very drinkable herb tea that is soothing and relaxing.*

Ready-made teabags

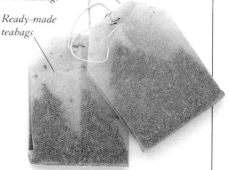

SALAD HERBS

FOR THE MEDIEVAL HOUSEWIFE a "green salad", made with highly-flavoured salad herbs and raw sliced vegetables, was a popular dish, that also acted as a springclean for digestions made sluggish by poor winter diet. Today, salad herbs are still widely appreciated for their beneficial properties. They have an extensive range of therapeutic actions: chicory is useful as a bile stimulant and laxative, fennel eases indigestion, watercress is a rich source of minerals and vitamins and cabbage – once known as the "poor man's medicine chest" – counters problems ranging from arthritis to threadworms.

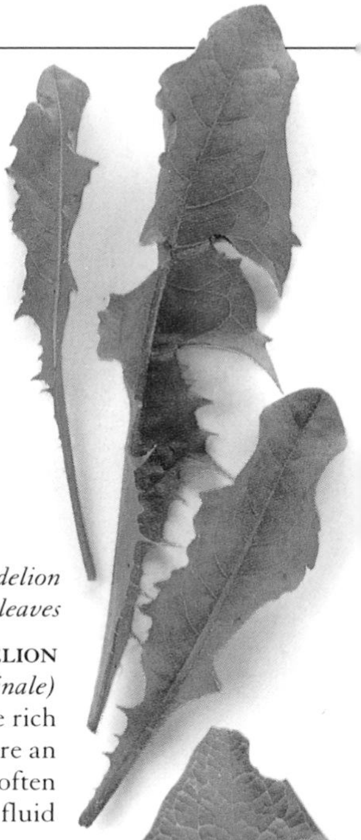

*Dandelion
leaves*

DANDELION
(*Taraxacum officinale*)
Dandelion leaves are rich in potassium. They are an effective diuretic, often used for fluid retention, as well as being a useful liver and digestive tonic.

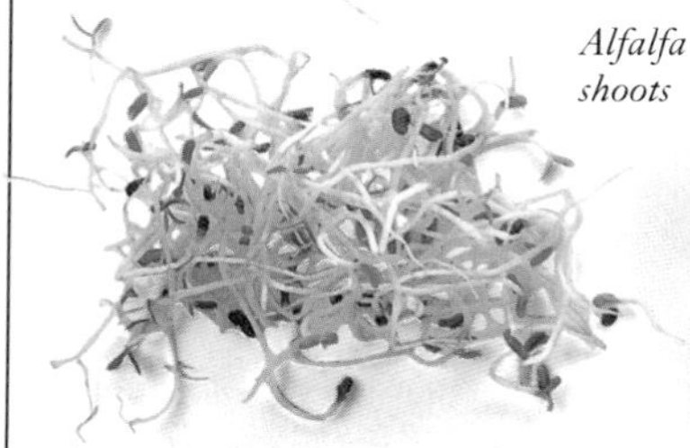

*Alfalfa
shoots*

ALFALFA (*Medicago sativa*)
Sprouted alfalfa is rich in calcium, magnesium, phosphorus, potassium and almost all known vitamins. It is regarded as a cleansing blood purifier in Eastern medicine.

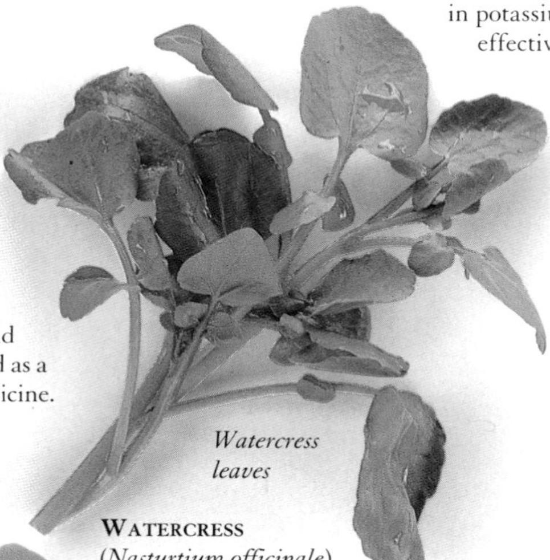

*Watercress
leaves*

WATERCRESS
(*Nasturtium officinale*)
Rich in minerals and vitamin C, watercress is an ideal tonic for anaemia.

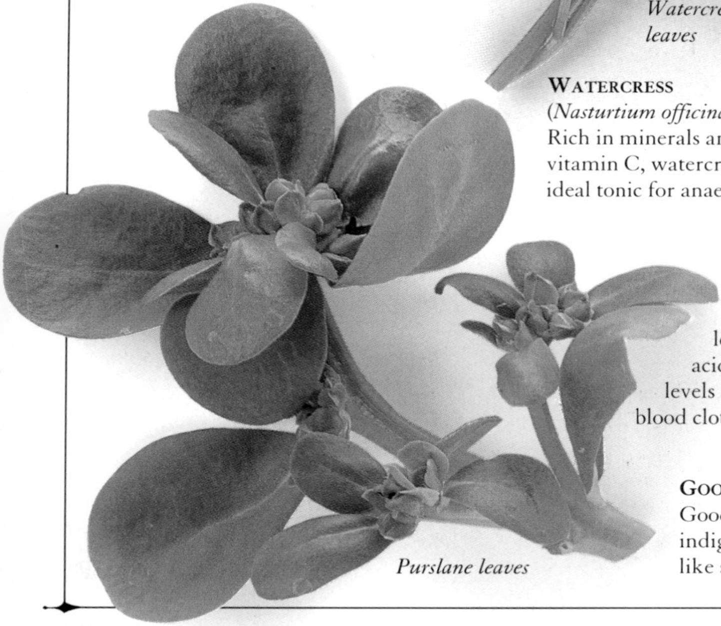

*Good King
Henry
leaves*

PURSLANE (*Portulaca oleracea*) Purslane is valued for its high level of omega-3 fatty acids, which affect cholesterol levels and reduce the risk of blood clots and heart attacks.

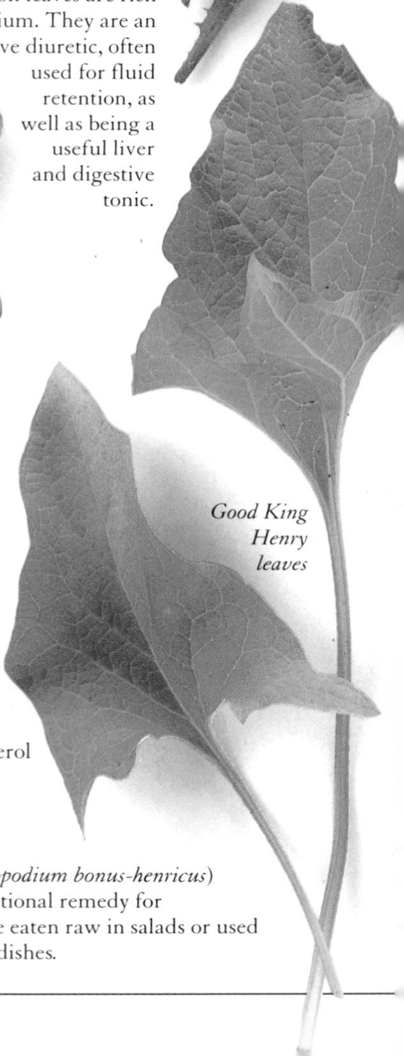

GOOD KING HENRY (*Chenopodium bonus-henricus*)
Good King Henry is a traditional remedy for indigestion. Its leaves can be eaten raw in salads or used like spinach in flans or egg dishes.

Purslane leaves

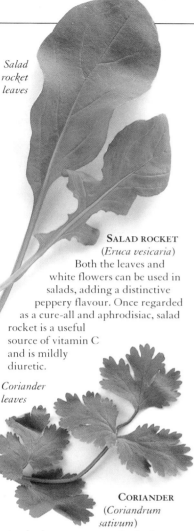

Salad rocket leaves

SALAD ROCKET
(*Eruca vesicaria*)
Both the leaves and
white flowers can be used in
salads, adding a distinctive
peppery flavour. Once regarded
as a cure-all and aphrodisiac, salad
rocket is a useful
source of vitamin C
and is mildly
diuretic.

Coriander leaves

CORIANDER
(*Coriandrum sativum*)
Coriander leaves are a popular Indian
household remedy for digestive upsets
and urinary tract infections.

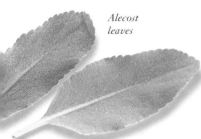

Alecost leaves

ALECOST, OR COSTMARY (*Tanacetum balsamita*) Alecost has astringent
properties and is used as a gentle digestive
stimulant. *Caution*: Do not confuse with the
camphor plant, which has similar leaves.

Salad recipes

Salad leaves, vegetables and herbs can be used in all kinds of combinations to make salads that will provide a beneficial addition to meals. Use ordinary lettuce as a base, or for a splash of colour, try chicory, lollo rosso, red cabbage or red orache. Then add salad herbs to suit your taste or dietary needs. Salad herbs are often highly flavoured and need to be used in moderation, especially if you are unfamiliar with the taste. Limit the use of strong digestive stimulants, such as dandelion, chicory or nasturtium if eating large amounts of salad.

TONIC SALAD

This mix contains herbs that stimulate the liver and adrenal glands and also provide plenty of vitamins and minerals.

~ HOW TO MAKE THE SALAD ~

Use lettuce – cos or little gem varieties if possible – and a few alfalfa sprouts. Add the following leaves roughly shredded: basil, dandelion, good King Henry and parsley. Toss in an olive oil and lemon juice dressing and decorate with nasturtium and borage flowers or chive florettes.

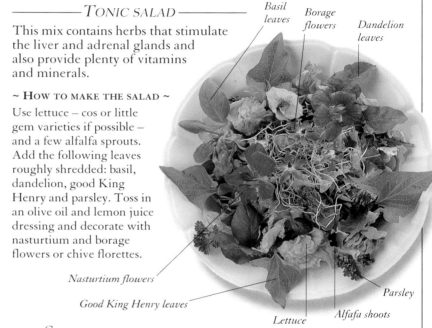

Basil leaves — *Borage flowers* — *Dandelion leaves* — *Parsley* — *Alfafa shoots* — *Lettuce* — *Good King Henry leaves* — *Nasturtium flowers*

SALAD FOR THE DIGESTION

This salad combines carminative herbs, used for easing indigestion, with gentle bile stimulants that give a mild laxative effect to help regulate the digestive system.

~ HOW TO MAKE THE SALAD ~

Finely slice a fennel bulb and combine with chicory leaves. Add 1–2 shredded alecost leaves and a small handful of lemon balm leaves. Toss in a dressing made from olive oil and lemon juice and decorate with sesame seeds or rocket flowers.

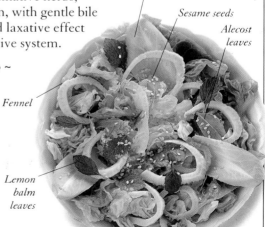

Chicory leaves — *Sesame seeds* — *Alecost leaves* — *Fennel* — *Lemon balm leaves*

MAKING HERBAL REMEDIES

Equipment

■ Use utensils made from cast iron, enamel, glass, pottery or stainless steel. Use wooden or steel spatulas and palette knives, and plastic or nylon sieves and tea strainers. Do not use aluminium pans, as many foods and herbs absorb this element, which is potentially toxic. Do not store herbal preparations in plastic containers for long periods, as plastic tends to absorb reactive chemicals from many herbs.
■ All equipment should be kept clean and storage bottles should be sterilized before use. If regularly making herbal remedies, keep a separate set of utensils for the purpose, to avoid contamination with food bacteria. Otherwise wash everything in very hot water and thoroughly dry all metal pans and spatulas in a hot oven before use. In addition, keep a separate teapot for making herbal infusions.
■ For equipment suppliers, see p. 140.
■ Label all ingredients and remedies clearly.

Weighing & measuring

WEIGHING HERBS Kitchen scales are generally suitable for weighing herbs. Electronic ones are the simplest to use, usually accurate to 0.1 g. If it is difficult to weigh less than 10 g on your scales, double the quantities given for dried herbs in a recipe and divide the mix in half, reserving one half for the next day's use.

MEASURING LIQUIDS Conical or straight-sided measuring cylinders are simple to use (see p. 74). If it is difficult to measure very small amounts of liquid try using a dropper. Twenty drops from a pipette equals approximately 1 ml.

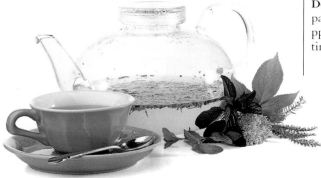

Sterilizing equipment

Many herbal medicines will soon go mouldy if non-sterile storage jars and bottles are used. There is rarely a problem with tinctures as the high alcohol content kills bacteria, but creams and syrups can rapidly deteriorate.

Sterilization preparations sold for home wine-making or for baby's bottles – usually based on sodium metabisulphite or sodium hypochlorite – are ideal. Before use, soak all storage bottles, jars and lids in a dilute mixture for at least 30 minutes (or as directed on the pack) and then rinse with freshly boiled water and dry in a hot oven.

Alternatively, wash glass containers thoroughly in freshly boiled water and place in a hot oven (at least 160° C/ 325° F/gas mark 3) for an hour. Handle with care when removing and use when cool. (This is not suitable for plastic containers.)

Cautions

COLLECTING PLANTS If using freshly gathered wild plant material to make herbal remedies, ensure that you have the correct plant by using a botanical field guide, as some plants may be confused: foxglove leaf, for example, is commonly mistaken for comfrey, and alkanet for borage. See also p. 135 for plants to handle with care.

ESSENTIAL OILS Commercially produced essential oils are commonly adulterated with cheap synthetic ingredients. When buying essential oils always opt for a reputable brand name. Do not take essential oils internally unless directed to do so by a professional practitioner.

DOSAGE The standard adult dose given on the following pages must be reduced for children and the elderly. See pp. 128 and 83 for advice. If pregnant, do not take alcoholic tinctures and see the list of herbs to avoid on p. 126.

MEASURING REMEDIES

1 ml = 20 drops	20 ml = 1 tablespoon
5 ml = 1 teaspoon	60–75 ml = 1 sherry glass
10 ml = 1 dessertspoon	150 ml =1 teacup or wineglass

SYRUPS

HONEY OR UNREFINED SUGAR can be combined with infusions or decoctions to make syrups. As well as helping to preserve the active plant ingredients, the sweetness is useful for disguising the flavour of some herbs, such as goldenseal, and syrups are frequently added to children's medicines. Honey has a particularly soothing effect and is often combined with herbs with an expectorant action to make cough syrups.

EQUIPMENT

• Teapot • Saucepan • Nylon or plastic sieve • Jug • Wooden spoon • Airtight, sterilized, dark glass bottles with cork stoppers • Funnel (optional)

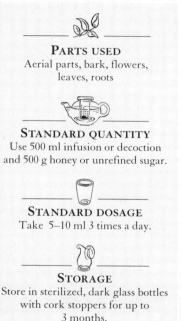

PARTS USED
Aerial parts, bark, flowers, leaves, roots

STANDARD QUANTITY
Use 500 ml infusion or decoction and 500 g honey or unrefined sugar.

STANDARD DOSAGE
Take 5–10 ml 3 times a day.

STORAGE
Store in sterilized, dark glass bottles with cork stoppers for up to 3 months.

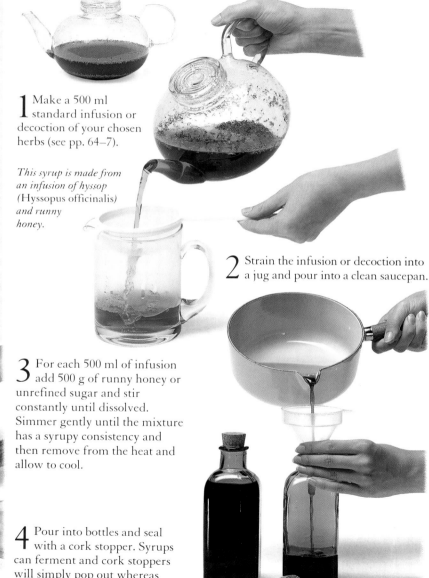

1 Make a 500 ml standard infusion or decoction of your chosen herbs (see pp. 64–7).

This syrup is made from an infusion of hyssop (Hyssopus officinalis) and runny honey.

2 Strain the infusion or decoction into a jug and pour into a clean saucepan.

3 For each 500 ml of infusion add 500 g of runny honey or unrefined sugar and stir constantly until dissolved. Simmer gently until the mixture has a syrupy consistency and then remove from the heat and allow to cool.

4 Pour into bottles and seal with a cork stopper. Syrups can ferment and cork stoppers will simply pop out whereas screw-top bottles can explode.

INFUSIONS

A VERY SIMPLE way of using herbs, infusions may be taken as remedies for specific ailments or be enjoyed generally, as relaxing and revitalizing teas. An infusion is made in a very similar way to tea, using fresh or dried herbs. The water should be just off the boil, as vigorously boiling water disperses valuable volatile oils in the steam. Infusions can be made from a single herb or from a combination of herbs, and may be drunk hot or cold. It is best to make them fresh each day.

EQUIPMENT
•*Kettle* • *Glass or ceramic teapot that holds at least 500 ml water*
• *Nylon or plastic tea strainer* • *Teacup*
• *Teaspoon* • *Jug with a lid for storage*

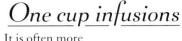

One cup infusions
It is often more convenient to make a single cup of infusion. These are made either in a small teapot or in a tisane cup (featured here), which are available from specialist outlets.

Lid

Stra

Cup

Saucer

PARTS USED
Leaves, flowers and most aerial parts (dried or fresh)

STANDARD QUANTITY
For most medicinal teas with a therapeutic action, add 25 g dried or 75 g fresh herb to 500 ml water to make 3 doses. If using a combination of herbs, ensure that the total weight of the mixture does not exceed the standard quantity.

STANDARD DOSAGE
Take a teacup or wineglass dose 3 times daily. Repeat doses may be reheated. Add a little honey or unrefined sugar per dose to taste. Reduce the dose for children and the elderly (see pp. 128 & 83).

STORAGE
Store in a covered jug in a cool place or refrigerator for up to 48 hours.

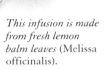

This infusion is made from fresh lemon balm leaves (Melissa officinalis).

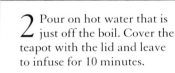

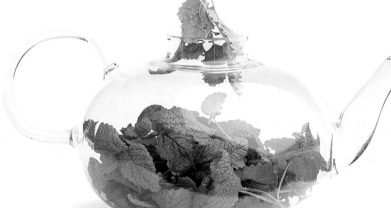

1 Warm a teapot with hot water. Add the fresh or dried herb.

2 Pour on hot water that is just off the boil. Cover the teapot with the lid and leave to infuse for 10 minutes.

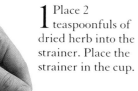

1 Place 2 teaspoonfuls of dried herb into the strainer. Place the strainer in the cup.

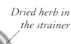

Dried herb in the strainer

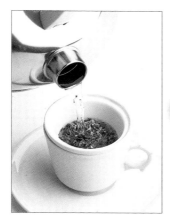

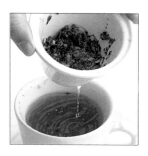

2 Pour freshly boiled water on to the herbs. Put the lid on and leave the tea to infuse for 10 minutes. Carefully remove the strainer.

Herbal teabags

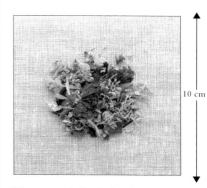

10 cm

4 Take a dose, adding honey or a little unrefined sugar to taste. Strain the rest into a jug, cover and store in a cool place or refrigerator.

Home-made herbal teabags are very useful when travelling or at the office. Place 1–2 teaspoons of herbs on a muslin square and tie it into a small bundle with string. Simply infuse this for 10 minutes in a teacup of freshly boiled water.

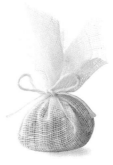

3 Strain the infusion through a tea strainer.

DECOCTIONS

THE DECOCTION METHOD is used for tough plant materials, such as barks, berries or roots, that need rather more vigorous extraction than is possible using the infusion method. Decoction involves heating the plant material in cold water, bringing it to the boil and simmering for 20–40 minutes. Combinations of herbs can be mixed together, or herbs may be used singly. The standard quantity should be made fresh each day, and is enough for three doses, which can be drunk hot or cold. As with infusions, decoctions are frequently used as the basis of other remedies, such as syrups.

EQUIPMENT
- *Saucepan (preferably ceramic, earthenware, enamel or stainless steel – do not use aluminium)*
- *Nylon or plastic sieve*
- *Jug with a lid for storage*

PARTS USED
Bark, berries, roots (dried or fresh)

STANDARD QUANTITY
Add 30 g dried or 60 g fresh herb to 750 ml of cold water. This reduces to around 500 ml after simmering. If using a combination of herbs, ensure that the total weight of the mixture does not exceed this standard amount.

STANDARD DOSAGE
Take a teacup or wineglass dose 3 times daily. Repeat doses may be reheated. Honey or unrefined sugar may be used to sweeten each dose, or they may be flavoured with a little lemon juice. Reduce the dose for children and the elderly (see pp. 128 & 83).

STORAGE
Store in a covered jug in a cool place or refrigerator for up to 48 hours.

Liquorice root

Gao Ben

Devil's claw

This decoction is made from dried liquorice root (Glycyrrhiza uralensis), *dried Gao Ben* (Ligusticum sinense) *and dried devil's claw* (Harpagophytum procumbens) .

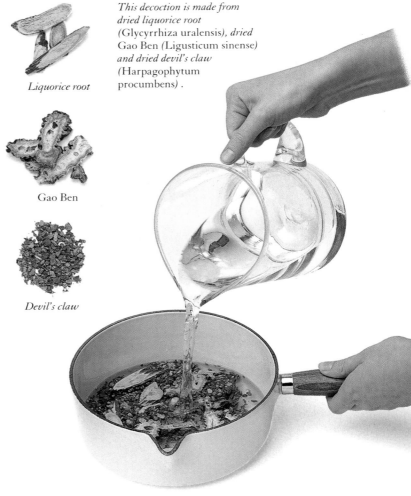

1 Place the herb in a saucepan and pour over the cold water.

2 Bring to the boil and simmer gently for 20–40 minutes, until the volume has reduced by about one-third.

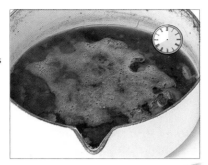

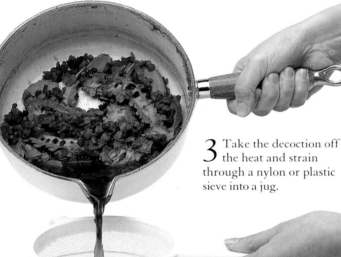

3 Take the decoction off the heat and strain through a nylon or plastic sieve into a jug.

4 Pour the decoction into a covered jug and store in a cool place or refrigerator.

Mixed decoction/infusion

For remedies that combine bark, berries or roots with flowers or leaves, use the following method.

1 Mix the bark, berries or roots together in a cast iron, stainless steel or enamel saucepan, and pour over 750 ml of cold water.

2 Bring to the boil, and simmer for 20–40 minutes, or until the volume has reduced by approximately one-third, to make a decoction.

3 Meanwhile, mix the flowers and leaves needed for the remedy and put them in a glass or ceramic teapot.

4 Strain the hot decoction on to the dried herbs in the teapot and leave to infuse for 10–15 minutes.

5 Strain the final mixture into a covered jug and store in a cool place. Take a teacup dose 3 times a day. Sweeten with a little honey or unrefined sugar to taste.

Macerations

There are some herbs, such as valerian root (*Valeriana officinalis*), that are best macerated rather than infused or decocted. Put 25 g of the dried herb in a saucepan. Add 500 ml of cold water and leave in a cool place overnight. Strain through a sieve.

Chinese decoctions

In China, herbs are mainly given in decoctions, and they tend to be more highly concentrated than in the West. Up to 150 g of dried herb to a litre of water is used, reduced down to 300–400 ml for 3 doses. The resulting mixture may need to be diluted with water to suit Western palates.

TINCTURES

TINCTURES ARE MADE BY steeping the herb in a mixture of alcohol and water. They should be made individually and prepared tinctures may then be combined as required. As well as extracting the plant's active ingredients, the alcohol acts as a preservative and tinctures will keep for up to two years. The liquid is usually composed of 25% alcohol and 75% water, but for some resinous herbs the amount of alcohol is increased to 45%. Commercially prepared tinctures use ethyl alcohol, but diluted spirits are suitable for home use. Vodka is ideal as it does not contain additives, but rum helps to disguise the flavour of less palatable herbs.

TINCTURE RATIOS *Tinctures are sometimes recommended for use in ratio form, for example, "take 5 ml of a 1:4 tincture". When making a tincture in ratio form, the proportion used is weight to volume. A 1:4 tincture could be made with 1 kg herb to 4 litres alcohol/water mix, or 100 g herb to 400 ml alcohol/water mix. The units used are immaterial and can be large or small accordingly.*

EQUIPMENT
- *Measuring jug* • *Large screw-top jar*
- *Muslin bag* • *Wine press*
- *Large jug* • *Sterilized, dark glass bottles with screw caps for airtight storage*
- *Funnel (optional)*

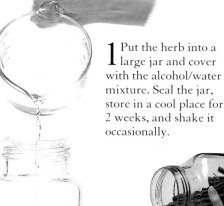

1 Put the herb into a large jar and cover with the alcohol/water mixture. Seal the jar, store in a cool place for 2 weeks, and shake it occasionally.

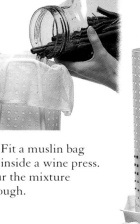

This tincture is made from cinnamon sticks (Cinnamomum zeylanicum) and a mixture of vodka and water.

PARTS USED
All parts of the plant (dried or fresh)

STANDARD QUANTITY
Use 200 g dried or 600 g fresh herb to 1 litre of alcohol/water mixture (25% alcohol & 75% water – e.g. dilute a 1 litre bottle of 37.5% vodka with 500 ml water). See Caution on p. 69 for types of alcohol not to use.

STANDARD DOSAGE
Take 5 ml 3 times a day diluted in a little warm water. A small amount of honey or fruit juice can often improve the flavour. See also Alcohol-reduced tinctures opposite.

STORAGE
Store in dark glass bottles for up to 2 years.

2 Fit a muslin bag inside a wine press. Pour the mixture through.

3 Press the mixture through the wine press into a jug. The residue can be added to the garden compost heap.

Alcohol-reduced tinctures

There are times when giving tinctures made from alcohol in the normal way is unsuitable, for example in pregnancy, in gastric or liver inflammation, or when treating children or reformed alcoholics. Adding a small amount (25–50 ml) of almost boiling water to the tincture dose (usually 5 ml) in a cup and allowing it to cool effectively evaporates most of the alcohol, making it safe.

CAUTIONS

- *Industrial alcohol, methylated spirits (methyl alcohol) and rubbing alcohol (isopropyl alcohol) are all extremely toxic. Do not use in tincture making.*
- *See Alcohol-reduced tinctures (above) for advice on giving tinctures to children, pregnant women and ex-alcoholics.*

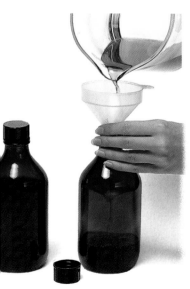

4 Pour the strained liquid into sterilized, dark glass bottles, using a funnel if necessary.

TONIC WINES

TONIC HERBS STEEPED IN WINE and taken in small, daily doses are used in many parts of the world as regular restoratives. Some commonly used in this way are the Chinese tonic herbs *Dang Gui, Dang Shen, He Shou Wu* and Korean ginseng. Western herbs, such as elecampane – a good lung tonic for those prone to coughs – can also be used. The easiest way to make a tonic wine is with a vinegar vat, which is a large ceramic pot with a tap at the bottom, allowing the liquid to be drained off easily. The herbs should always be kept covered with wine, or they may go mouldy and the mixture will have to be discarded.

EQUIPMENT

- *Vinegar vat* • *Alternatively use a jug with a well fitting lid and pour the daily dose from the top of the mixture, ensuring it is regularly stirred.*

This tonic wine is made with dried Dang Gui *(Chinese angelica – Angelica sinensis) and red wine.*

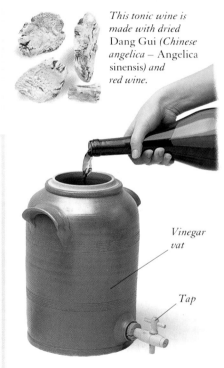

Vinegar vat

Tap

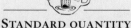

PARTS USED
Roots (dried)

STANDARD QUANTITY
Add enough dried herb to fill the vinegar vat at least three-quarters full and good quality red or white wine to cover the herb completely. Additional wine will be needed to top up the vat.

STANDARD DOSAGE
Take a sherry-glass dose daily.

STORAGE
The tonic wine may be kept for 3–4 months if regularly topped up. Throw the mixture away if the herbs go mouldy and start again.

1 Fill the vat at least three-quarters full with the chosen herb. Pour on enough wine to cover the mixture completely.

2 Leave for 2 weeks, then take a daily dose from the tap at the bottom of the vat. Make sure the herbs always remain covered with wine and top up the vat regularly.

CAPSULES

HERBS CAN BE TAKEN IN POWDERED form: sprinked on food, stirred in water or made into capsules, which are preferable for the less palatable herbs as well as convenient for carrying around. It is best to use commercially produced powders, available from specialist suppliers (see p. 140). Two-part gelatin or vegetarian capsules may also be obtained from specialist outlets.

(see p. 140)

EQUIPMENT

- *Saucer or flat dish*
- *Capsule cases* • *Dark, airtight containers for storage*

PARTS USED
All parts of the plant
(dried and powdered)

STANDARD QUANTITY
Use 200–250 mg powder to each size
00 gelatin or vegetarian capsule case.

STANDARD DOSAGE
Take 2–3 capsules 2 to 3 times a day.

STORAGE
Store in airtight, dark containers in
a cool place for up to 3–4 months.

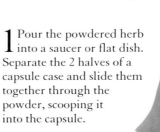

The capsules are filled with powdered ginger (Zingiber officinalis).

1 Pour the powdered herb into a saucer or flat dish. Separate the 2 halves of a capsule case and slide them together through the powder, scooping it into the capsule.

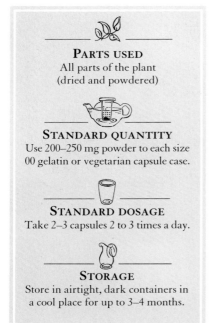

2 Fit together the 2 halves of the capsule. Store in dark, airtight containers in a cool place.

PESSARIES & SUPPOSITORIES

PESSARIES ARE WAXY pellets containing medication. They are inserted in the vagina and melt at body temperature, delivering the remedy to the site of infection or irritation. Suppositories are similar but intended for anal insertion. They are used when treatments are needed in the lower bowel and medicines taken orally would be broken down during the digestive process. It is best to buy them ready-made. To make pessaries:

1 Use a pessary mould (available from specialist suppliers) or make 24 suitable shapes from cooking foil (1 cm in diameter tapering to 0.5 cm in diameter at one end, and 2 cm in length). Place them on a wire grill. Combine 10 g soft soap, 50 ml glycerine and 40 ml methylated spirits to make a lubricant and pour into the mould or shapes. Leave for a few seconds and pour away.

2 Melt 20 g cocoa butter in a double saucepan. Remove the pan from the heat and add 30 drops of essential oil. Pour the mixture into the moulds and leave to set for about 3 hours. When fully set, open the mould or carefully remove the cooking foil.

3 Store the pessaries in a cool place in a pot lined with greaseproof paper.

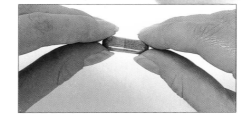

Marigold & thyme pessaries

COMPRESSES

A COMPRESS IS A cloth soaked in a hot or cold herbal extract. They can be applied to painful joints and muscles and are useful for soothing skin rashes and irritations. A cold compress is sometimes used for headaches. The cloth may be soaked in an infusion, decoction or a tincture diluted with hot or cold water. A tea towel is ideal, or use muslin or cottonwool wrapped in surgical gauze.

EQUIPMENT
• *Cloth pad* • *Bowl*

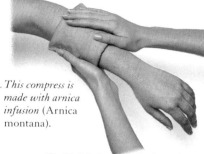

This compress is made with arnica infusion (Arnica montana).

STANDARD QUANTITY
Use 500 ml standard infusion or decoction, or 50 ml tincture in 500 ml hot or cold water.

STANDARD APPLICATION
Apply as often as required.

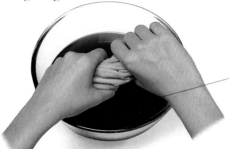

1 Soak a clean piece of soft cloth in a hot infusion or other herbal extract. Squeeze out the excess liquid.

2 Hold the pad against the affected area. When it cools or dries, repeat the process using hot mixture.

POULTICES

A POULTICE OF BREAD or mashed potato soaked in herbal extract was once a favourite household remedy for minor injuries and ailments. Today, poultices are generally made with chopped fresh herbs. They are generally applied hot.

EQUIPMENT
• *Saucepan* • *Gauze/cotton strips*

This poultice is made with fresh chopped cabbage leaves (Brassica oleracea).

PARTS USED
Whole plant (dried or fresh) chopped

STANDARD QUANTITY
Use sufficient herb to cover the area.

STANDARD APPLICATION
Apply the poultice every 2–4 hours or more frequently if necessary.

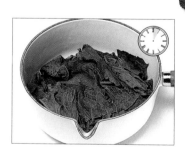

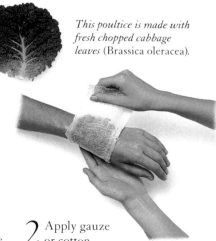

1 Boil the fresh herb, squeeze out any surplus liquid and spread it on to the affected area. Smooth a little oil on the skin first, to prevent the herb sticking.

2 Apply gauze or cotton strips to hold the poultice in place.

HOT INFUSED OILS

ACTIVE PLANT INGREDIENTS can be extracted in oil for external use in massage oils, creams and ointments. Infused oils will last for up to a year if kept in a cool, dark place, but they are more potent when fresh, so it is best to make small amounts frequently. There are two techniques for making infused oils and the hot method is suitable for leafy herbs such as comfrey, chickweed, stinging nettle and rosemary.

This hot infused oil [is] made with dried chickweed (Stellaria media).

EQUIPMENT
• *Glass bowl and saucepan, or double saucepan* • *Muslin bag and wine press (or jelly bag)* • *Large jug* • *Airtight, sterilized, dark glass storage bottles* • *Funnel (optional)*

PARTS USED
Aerial parts, leaves (dried)

STANDARD QUANTITY
Use 250 g dried herb to 500 ml sunflower oil.

STORAGE
Store in sterilized, airtight dark glass bottles in a cool place away from direct light for up to a year.

Suitable herbs

Herbs used to make hot infused oils include:
• *Bladderwrack* for arthritic pain.
• *Chickweed* for irritant eczema.
• *Cleavers* for psoriasis.
• *Comfrey* for bruises, sprains and osteoarthritis.
• *Stinging nettle* for allergic skin rashes and eczema.
• *Rosemary* for aches and pains.

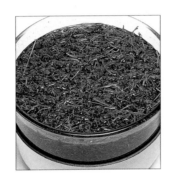

1 Put the oil and the herb in a glass bowl over a pan of simmering water or in a double saucepan and heat gently for about 3 hours.

Muslin bag

Wine press

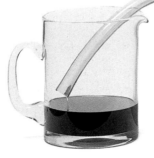

2 Strain the mixture through a muslin bag fitted to a wine press into a jug. Alternatively, strain it through a jelly bag (illustrated on p. 73).

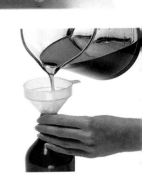

3 Pour the oil into storage bottles, using a funnel if necessary.

COLD INFUSED OILS

THIS METHOD OF MAKING AN infused oil is suitable for flowers such as pot marigold and St John's wort. It is a slow process: the flowers and oil are packed into a jar and left for several weeks, after which the once-infused oil is used again with fresh herb to extract as much active plant ingredient as possible. Cold infused oils are used in massage oils or as the basis of creams or ointments – see below for herbs commonly used in this way.

EQUIPMENT

Large glass screw-top jar • Jelly bag and string (or muslin bag and wine press) • Large jug • Airtight, sterilized, dark glass storage bottles • Funnel (optional)

PARTS USED

Aerial parts, flowers (fresh or dried)

STANDARD QUANTITY

Use double quantities of enough fresh or dried herb to pack a storage jar, and about 1 litre cold-pressed safflower or walnut oil (the quantity will depend on the size of jar used).

STORAGE

Store in sterilized, airtight dark glass bottles in a cool place away from direct light for up to a year.

Suitable herbs

Herbs used to make cold infused oils include:
- *Melilot* (use dried herb) for varicose eczema.
- *Pot marigold* (use fresh or dried petals) for grazes, dry eczema and fungal infections such as thrush and athlete's foot.
- *St John's wort* (use fresh flowering tops) for sunburn, minor scalds and burns, grazes and inflamed joints.

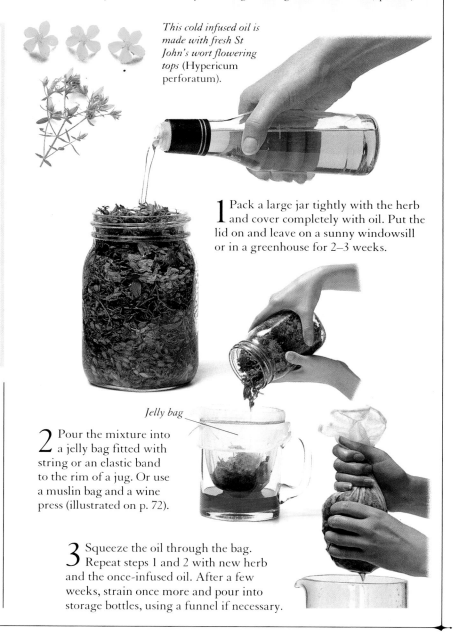

This cold infused oil is made with fresh St John's wort flowering tops (Hypericum perforatum).

1 Pack a large jar tightly with the herb and cover completely with oil. Put the lid on and leave on a sunny windowsill or in a greenhouse for 2–3 weeks.

Jelly bag

2 Pour the mixture into a jelly bag fitted with string or an elastic band to the rim of a jug. Or use a muslin bag and a wine press (illustrated on p. 72).

3 Squeeze the oil through the bag. Repeat steps 1 and 2 with new herb and the once-infused oil. After a few weeks, strain once more and pour into storage bottles, using a funnel if necessary.

MASSAGE OILS

MASSAGE OILS ARE MADE from a few drops of essential oil diluted in a carrier oil – sweet almond or wheatgerm is best, but sunflower or other vegetable oil may be used. Infused oils are also used as carriers. Once diluted, essential oils soon deteriorate, so it is best to mix small amounts frequently. Massage requires skill and practice, and is not suitable for some conditions (see Cautions below).

EQUIPMENT
- *Small and large measuring cylinders*
- *50 ml sterilized, airtight dark glass bottle • Funnel (optional)*

PARTS USED
Essential oil

STANDARD QUANTITY
In general, use no more than a 10% concentration of essential oils i.e. up to 5 ml of essential oil in 45 ml of carrier oil (sweet almond, wheatgerm or vegetable oil). Reduce this to a maximum of 5% essential oil for children, the elderly or those with sensitive skins. Use good quality essential oil.

STANDARD APPLICATION
Pour about 2–5 ml (½–1 teaspoonful) on to the hands (not directly on to the body) and rub gently.

STORAGE
Store in a sterilized, airtight dark glass bottle in a cool place.

CAUTIONS FOR MASSAGE
- *Pregnant women should seek professional advice and should not use essential oil at all during the first 3 months of pregnancy.*
- *Do not massage anyone suffering from an infection, epilepsy, a contagious disease, acute back pain (especially if the pain shoots down the arms and legs), or from an inflammatory condition such as thrombosis or phlebitis.*
- *Do not massage bruised or inflamed areas.*

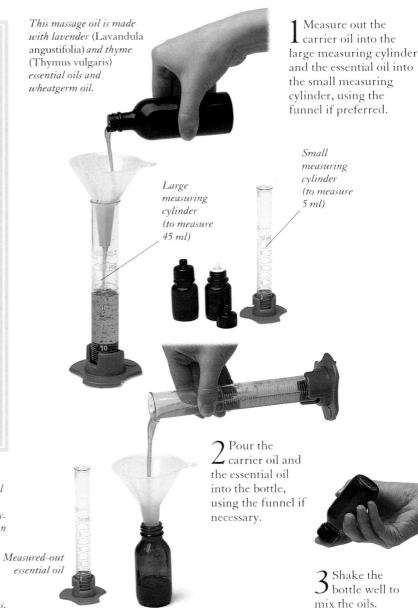

This massage oil is made with lavender (Lavandula angustifolia) and thyme (Thymus vulgaris) essential oils and wheatgerm oil.

1 Measure out the carrier oil into the large measuring cylinder and the essential oil into the small measuring cylinder, using the funnel if preferred.

Large measuring cylinder (to measure 45 ml)

Small measuring cylinder (to measure 5 ml)

2 Pour the carrier oil and the essential oil into the bottle, using the funnel if necessary.

Measured-out essential oil

3 Shake the bottle well to mix the oils.

OINTMENTS

OINTMENTS CONTAIN oils or fats, but no water, and unlike creams, they do not blend with the skin, but form a separate layer over it. They are suitable where the skin is already weak or soft, or where some protection is needed from additional moisture, as in nappy rash. Ointments were once made from animal fats, but petroleum jelly or paraffin wax is suitable. Infused oils may be used instead of the herb itself (see p. 76).

(see p. 76)

EQUIPMENT

• *Glass bowl and saucepan, or double saucepan* • *Wooden spoon* • *Jelly bag and string (or muslin bag and wine press)* • *Jug* • *Rubber gloves* • *Sterilized, airtight dark glass jars with lids*

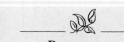

PARTS USED
All parts of the plant (dried and fresh)

STANDARD QUANTITY
Use 500 g petroleum jelly or soft paraffin wax and 60 g dried or 150 g fresh herb.

STANDARD APPLICATION
Rub a little into the affected part 2–3 times a day.

STORAGE
Store in sterilized, airtight dark jars, in a cool place for 3–4 months.

This ointment is made with dried stinging nettle (Urtica dioica).

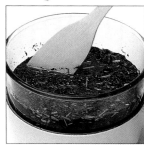

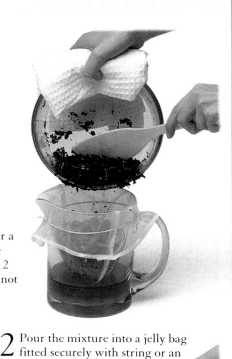

1 Melt the jelly or wax in a bowl over a pan of boiling water or in a double saucepan. Add the herbs and heat for 2 hours or until the herbs are crisp. Do not allow the pan to boil dry.

Suitable herbs

• *Arnica* for bruises, sprains and chilblains (only use on unbroken skin).
• *Capsicum* for shingles.
• *Chamomile* for eczema and other allergic skin conditions.
• *Chickweed* for irritant eczema, corns, boils or splinters.
• *Elderflower* for chapped hands.
• *Heartsease* for rashes.
• *Melilot* for swellings and varicose eczema.
• *Plantain* for dry eczema.
Stinging nettle for haemorrhoids and eczema.

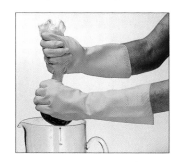

2 Pour the mixture into a jelly bag fitted securely with string or an elastic band to the rim of a jug. Or use a muslin bag and a wine press (see p. 72).

(see p. 72)

3 If using a jelly bag wear rubber gloves, as the mixture is hot. Squeeze the mixture through the jelly bag into the jug.

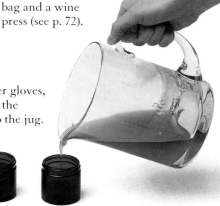

4 Quickly pour the strained mixture, while still warm and molten, into jars.

CREAMS

A CREAM IS A MIXTURE of water with fats or oils, which softens and blends with the skin. It can be easily made using emulsifying ointment (available from most pharmacies), which is a mixture of oils and waxes that blends with water or tinctures. Home-made creams will last for several months, but the shelf-life is prolonged by storing the mixture in a cool larder or refrigerator or by adding a few drops of benzoin tincture as a preservative. Creams made from organic oils and fats deteriorate more quickly. The method shown here is suitable for most herbs.

EQUIPMENT

Glass bowl and saucepan, or double saucepan • Wooden spoon or spatula • Wine press and muslin bag (or jelly bag and jug) • Bowl • Small palette knife • Small, sterilized, airtight, dark storage jars

PARTS USED
All parts of the plant
(fresh or dried)

STANDARD QUANTITY
Use 150 g emulsifying ointment,
70 ml glycerol, 80 ml water and
30 g dried or 75 g fresh herb.

STANDARD APPLICATION
Rub a little into the affected part
2–3 times a day.

STORAGE
Store in sterilized, airtight dark jars
in a cool place for up to 3 months.

This cream is made with dried pot marigold (Calendula officinalis).

1 Melt the emulsifying ointment in a double saucepan or a bowl over a pan of boiling water. Pour in the glycerol and water and stir well. The mixture will solidify slightly when the liquid is added, so keep the bowl over the boiling water and stir to re-melt it.

2 Add the herb and stir well. Simmer for 3 hours, regularly adding more boiling water to the lower saucepan to prevent the pan from burning.

3 Use a wine press, or jelly bag fitted to a jug and strain the hot mixture as quickly as possible into a bowl. Stir the molten, strained cream constantly as it cools, to avoid separation. If it does start to separate, return it to the double saucepan and reheat with an additional 10–20 g of emulsifying ointment.

CREAMS & OINTMENTS FROM INFUSED OILS
Creams and ointments can be made using hot and cold infused oils instead of dried herbs. (To make infused oils, see pp. 72–3.) For a cream, melt 25 g beeswax with 25 g anhydrous lanolin (both available over the counter), add 100 ml infused oil and 50 ml herbal tincture (to make, see p. 68). Strain, stir and when the cream has set, put into storage jars using a palette knife. To make an ointment, melt 25 g beeswax with 25 g anhydrous lanolin, then add 100 ml infused oil. Pour into sterilized, dark glass jars while still warm, and allow to cool.

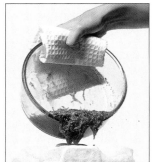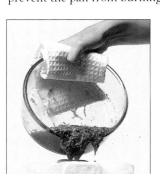

4 When the cream has set, use a small palette knife to fill storage jars. Put some cream around the edge of the jar first, and then fill the middle to avoid air bubbles.

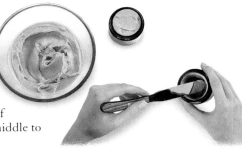

LOTIONS & EMULSIONS

A LOTION IS A WATER-BASED mixture, applied to the skin as a cooling or soothing remedy to relieve irritation or inflammation. Alcohol-based mixtures – such as tinctures – may be added to lotions to increase the cooling effect. Emulsions are also water-based mixtures, consisting of oil and water shaken to form a suspension. Both remedies are made in the same way and can be stored for up to three months.

EQUIPMENT

- *Measuring cylinder*
- *Sterilized, dark glass storage bottles*
- *Funnel (optional)*

PARTS USED
All parts of the plant
(fresh or dried)

STANDARD QUANTITY
Lotions and emulsions vary in composition depending on use. The lotion featured here is for an irritant skin rash: 40 ml distilled witch hazel, 40 ml rose water, 20 ml chickweed tincture. An emulsion for warts can be made by combining 5 ml tea tree oil and 5 ml thuja tincture.

STANDARD APPLICATION
Lotions and emulsions are usually mild and can be used liberally as required to ease symptoms.

STORAGE
Store in sterilized, dark glass bottles in a cool place for up to 3 months.

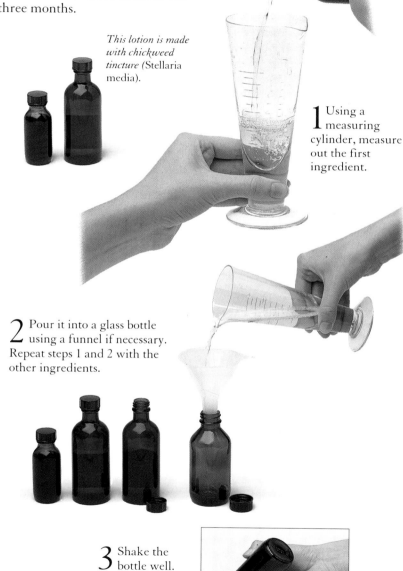

This lotion is made with chickweed tincture (Stellaria media).

1 Using a measuring cylinder, measure out the first ingredient.

2 Pour it into a glass bottle using a funnel if necessary. Repeat steps 1 and 2 with the other ingredients.

3 Shake the bottle well.

STEAM INHALATIONS

CONDITIONS SUCH AS catarrh, sinusitis, bronchitis or asthma can be relieved with steam inhalations, which clear the respiratory system of excess mucus. Well diluted infusions or essential oils are used, with active plant ingredients that are anti-allergenic and anti-inflammatory. After treatment, stay in a warm room for 30 minutes to allow the airways to readjust.

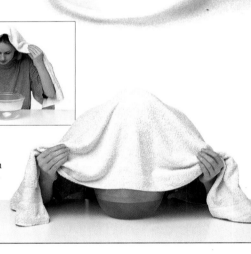

This steam inhalation uses chamomile essential oil (Matricaria recutita

EQUIPMENT
• *Kettle* • *Basin* • *Towel*

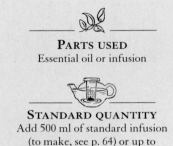

PARTS USED
Essential oil or infusion

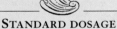

STANDARD QUANTITY
Add 500 ml of standard infusion (to make, see p. 64) or up to 10 drops of good quality essential oil (see the note on p. 62) to a basin of steaming hot water.

STANDARD DOSAGE
Use once or twice a day, inhaling the steam for 10 minutes each time.

1 Boil a kettle and half fill a basin with boiling water. Add 500 ml of standard infusion or 5–10 drops of essential oil (or a mixture of oils).

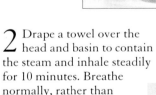

2 Drape a towel over the head and basin to contain the steam and inhale steadily for 10 minutes. Breathe normally, rather than too deeply.

BATHS & WASHES

ESSENTIAL OILS CAN BE added to bathwater for a relaxing soak, to ease aching limbs, clear stuffy noses and relieve many other minor ailments. Use 2–5 drops of essential oil neat in the bathwater and stir well to disperse the oil. Some of the more useful oils are:
• *Chamomile* for anxiety, insomnia and period pain.
• *Eucalyptus* for coughs, colds, aches and pains.
• *Lavender* for headaches, aches and pains, and stress.
• *Peppermint* for fatigue and nasal congestion.
• *Rosemary* for fatigue, aching joints and period pain.

Footbaths

Footbaths are ideal for relieving aching feet, easing sprains, or stimulating the circulation for those prone to chilblains. The traditional mustard bath, using a dessertspoon of powdered culinary mustard to a basin of hot water, is still an effective treatment today. In addition, hot and cold treatments can help reduce bruising and bring some relief for badly sprained ankles. Put the feet in a basin of very hot water containing a large handful of rosemary sprigs for 3–5 minutes and then plunge into a basin of iced water for 2–3 minutes. Repeat as many times as you can bear.

EYEBATHS

EYEBATHS ARE SIMPLE to make and use, and can be very soothing for a range of eye complaints. The mixtures should not sting at all – if they do, dilute further, as individual sensitivity can vary. Use weak infusions or decoctions or two drops of tincture to an eyebath filled with freshly boiled water. See the Caution right, about sterilizing the eyebath.

CAUTION

It is very important to sterilize the eyebath thoroughly (see p. 62) in between bathing each eye, especially in infectious conditions.

EQUIPMENT

• *Saucepan* • *Sieve* • *Jug* • *Eyebath*

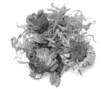

This eyebath is made with a decoction of pot marigold (Calendula officinalis) and eyebright (Euphrasia officinalis).

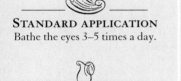

STANDARD QUANTITY

Use 400 ml decoction, made with 15 g dried herb and 600 ml water (see p. 66), or 400 ml infusion, made with 15 g dried herb and 500 ml water (see p. 64), or 2 drops of tincture (see p. 68) in an eyebath of freshly boiled water.

STANDARD APPLICATION

Bathe the eyes 3–5 times a day.

STORAGE

Store in a covered jug in a cool place. Make a fresh eyebath each day.

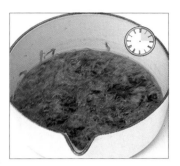

1 Make a decoction or infusion of your chosen herb. Simmer for 10–15 minutes to ensure sterility.

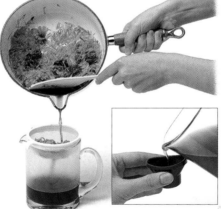

2 Strain well through a fine sieve. Ensure there are no particles of herb remaining that might irritate the eye.

3 Allow the mixture to cool to a lukewarm temperature and then fill an eyebath with the mixture.

4 Placing the eyebath over the eye, lean back so the eye is well wetted and blink several times.

GARGLES & MOUTHWASHES

GARGLES AND MOUTHWASHES can be made either from standard infusions and decoctions (to make, see pp. 64–7) or by diluting tinctures (to make, see p. 68). If using standard infusions or decoctions, strain well, allow the mixture to cool and use in wineglass doses. If using tinctures, dilute 5 ml of tincture in a wineglass of warm water. Herbs will carry on working as they are digested, so gargles and mouthwashes made in this way can be swallowed as standard infusions and tinctures would be.

OVER-THE-COUNTER REMEDI

THE DAYS WHEN HERBAL REMEDIES were only made at home are over. Today, the market in over-the-counter herbal products is huge – but choosing the right remedy is not always easy. In many countries, products are carefully regulated: in Europe, for example, herbal remedies are licensed and their efficacy must be proven before medical claims for them can be made. For legal reasons many remedies are not labelled with recommended medical uses, although their names may be suitably suggestive. If products and their actions are not clearly labelled, consumers should check the actions of individual herbs listed on the pack. It is always best to buy remedies from reputable suppliers with product licences or to choose remedies on the recommendation of a professional herbalist. Where it is given, consumers should follow the recommended dosage, otherwise check the dosage with a professional herbalist.

Tablets & capsules

Herbs are most commonly sold in easy-to-take tablets or capsules. Many suppliers will provide information and sell herb mixes recommended for self-limiting ailments. A list of herbs commonly found in tablets and capsules follows:

BLUE FLAG – *for minor skin problems.*
BOLDO – *a digestive stimulant and urinary antiseptic sometimes sold in remedies for cystitis.*
BORAGE OIL, OR STAR FLOWER OIL – *rich in gamma-linolenic acid; sold as a supplement for menstrual disorders and skin complaints.*

BURDOCK – *has a mild laxative action: promoted as a "spring cleaning" remedy.*
CASCARA – *a laxative; avoid when pregnant.*
CHASTEBERRY, OR AGNUS CASTUS – *usually recommended for various gynaecological problems; overdose can cause formication (a sensation of ants crawling on the skin).*
CRANESBILL – *an astringent herb often used in commercial diarrhoea remedies.*
DAMIANA – *sold as a general tonic and, sometimes, as an aphrodisiac.*
DANG GUI, OR TANG KWAI – *included as a tonic in specific women's remedies.*
DEVIL'S CLAW – *recommended for arthritis.*
ECHINACEA– *an immune stimulant for colds.*

EPHEDRA, OR MA HUANG – *often containe in patent sinusitis and catarrh remedies.*
EVENING PRIMROSE OIL – *rich in gamma-linolenic acid and marketed as a supplement for menstrual disorders and skin complaints.*
FENUGREEK – *used in digestive stimulants and milk-stimulants for breastfeeding mothers.*
FEVERFEW – *for migraines and rheumatism*
GARLIC – *used both as a cold cure and to help reduce cholesterol levels.*
GINGER – *used in travel sickness remedies.*
GINKGO – *a remedy for poor circulation.*
GINSENG – *a general purpose tonic.*
GOLDENSEAL – *a liver stimulant and anti-catarrhal, often sold as an indigestion remedy.*

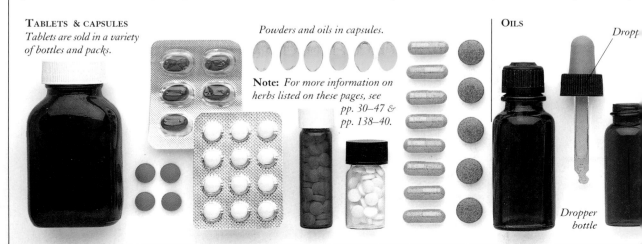

TABLETS & CAPSULES
Tablets are sold in a variety of bottles and packs.

Powders and oils in capsules.

Note: *For more information on herbs listed on these pages, see* pp. 30–47 & pp. 138–40.

OILS

Dropp

Dropper bottle

GOTU KOLA – *a tonic used in convalescence.*
GUARANA – *a general-purpose tonic.*
HELONIAS – *included in remedies for menstrual and menopausal problems.*
HE SHOU WU, OR FO TI – *a Chinese tonic herb used in some Western laxative mixtures but best regarded as a kidney tonic.*
HUANG QI, OR ASTRALAGUS ROOT *a popular Chinese tonic.*
KELP – *a metabolic stimulant.*
PAPAYA – *a digestive remedy.*
PARSLEY – *often included in diuretic mixtures for premenstrual fluid retention.*
PILEWORT – *sometimes sold for internal consumption for haemorrhoids.*
PSYLLIUM SEEDS, OR ISPHAGULA – *laxative.*
SENNA – *laxative: avoid in pregnancy.*
SLIPPERY ELM – *for digestive problems and sore throats.*
UVA-URSI – *used in many diuretic mixtures for premenstrual fluid retention.*
VALERIAN – *used in calming mixtures for insomnia or nervous tension.*

Oils

When buying essential oils, choose well-known, reputable brands as oils are prone to adulteration and synthetic substitution. Quality products will be more expensive. Check properties in a specialist aromatherapy guide and do not take essential oils internally except under professional direction.

Ointments & creams

Commercially available herbal ointments and creams tend to be limited to the most popular remedies. They may also be bought from suppliers of homeopathic and anthroposophical medicines under a variety of brand names. The following are commonly available:

ALOE VERA – *sold in cosmetic preparations but also valuable for sunburn and sores.*
ARNICA – *excellent for bruises and injuries but should not be used on broken skin.*
CALENDULA, OR POT MARIGOLD – *useful antiseptic and antifungal, helpful for dry skin conditions.*
CHICKWEED – *draws infections from wounds and eases irritant skin conditions.*
COMFREY – *a restricted herb in many countries but a valuable and safe remedy when used externally for bruises and strains.*
HYPERICUM, OR ST JOHN'S WORT – *often sold in combination with calendula for minor skin problems and burns.*
SAGE – *used for insect bites and as a general purpose skin remedy.*
TEA TREE – *potent antibacterial for grazes and skin infections.*
URTICA, OR STINGING NETTLE – *usually available from homeopathic suppliers for irritant skin conditions.*

Syrups, extracts & juices

Availability of liquid herbal extracts varies markedly between countries. In Germany, for example, a huge variety is available, largely supplied on prescription, while in other countries the range is more limited. Juices can sometimes be found in health food shops and can be taken singly or combined with tinctures or syrups. Few products give any details of the herbs' actions so check before taking. Among the more useful juices that may be found are:

ARTICHOKE – *a liver stimulant and digestive remedy.*
BLACK RADISH – *a digestive remedy.*
BORAGE – *useful to stimulate adrenal glands and also used externally for irritant rashes on the skin.*
HORSETAIL – *rich in silica and suitable for deep-seated lung problems.*
OATS – *a tonic nervine useful for depression.*
RAMSONS – *wild garlic, a milder form of the familiar herb used in a similar way – to combat colds and help the immune system.*
SILVERWEED – *an anticatarrhal member of the rose family which can be helpful for sinus problems.*

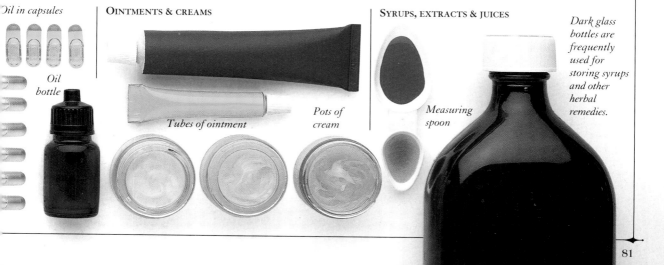

Oil in capsules

Oil bottle

OINTMENTS & CREAMS

Tubes of ointment

Pots of cream

SYRUPS, EXTRACTS & JUICES

Measuring spoon

Dark glass bottles are frequently used for storing syrups and other herbal remedies.

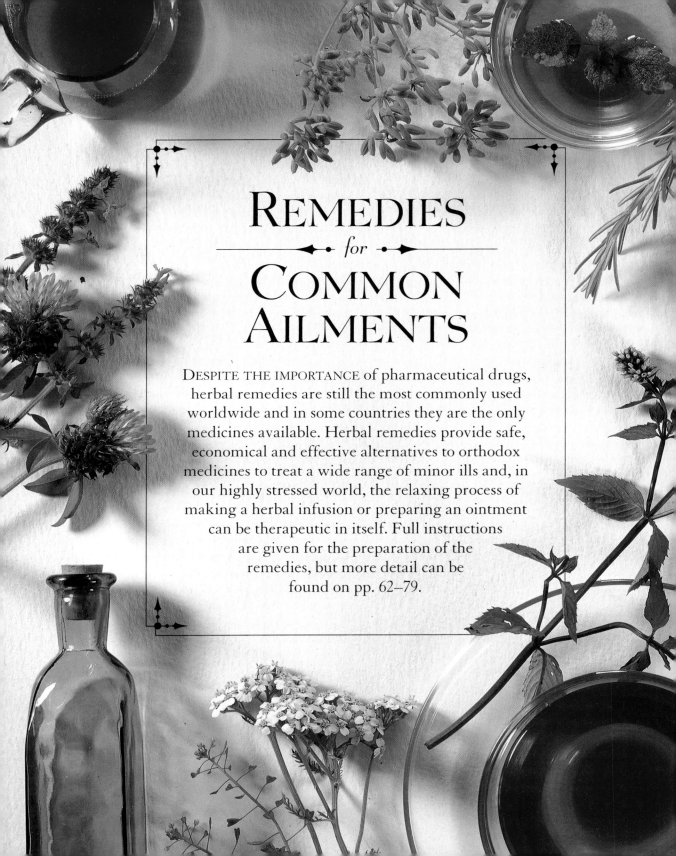

REMEDIES
for
COMMON AILMENTS

DESPITE THE IMPORTANCE of pharmaceutical drugs, herbal remedies are still the most commonly used worldwide and in some countries they are the only medicines available. Herbal remedies provide safe, economical and effective alternatives to orthodox medicines to treat a wide range of minor ills and, in our highly stressed world, the relaxing process of making a herbal infusion or preparing an ointment can be therapeutic in itself. Full instructions are given for the preparation of the remedies, but more detail can be found on pp. 62–79.

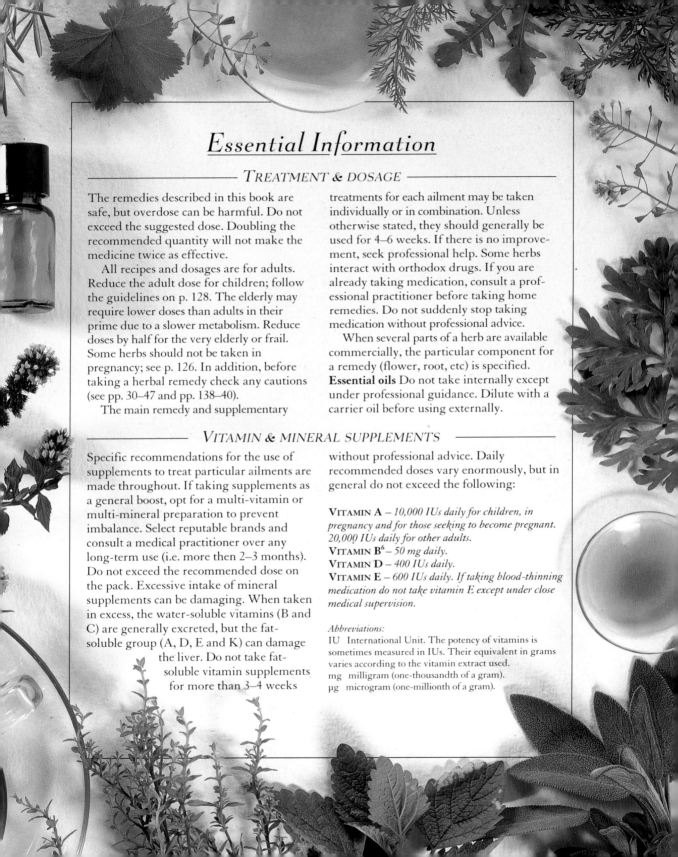

Essential Information

TREATMENT & DOSAGE

The remedies described in this book are safe, but overdose can be harmful. Do not exceed the suggested dose. Doubling the recommended quantity will not make the medicine twice as effective.

All recipes and dosages are for adults. Reduce the adult dose for children; follow the guidelines on p. 128. The elderly may require lower doses than adults in their prime due to a slower metabolism. Reduce doses by half for the very elderly or frail. Some herbs should not be taken in pregnancy; see p. 126. In addition, before taking a herbal remedy check any cautions (see pp. 30–47 and pp. 138–40).

The main remedy and supplementary treatments for each ailment may be taken individually or in combination. Unless otherwise stated, they should generally be used for 4–6 weeks. If there is no improvement, seek professional help. Some herbs interact with orthodox drugs. If you are already taking medication, consult a professional practitioner before taking home remedies. Do not suddenly stop taking medication without professional advice.

When several parts of a herb are available commercially, the particular component for a remedy (flower, root, etc) is specified. **Essential oils** Do not take internally except under professional guidance. Dilute with a carrier oil before using externally.

VITAMIN & MINERAL SUPPLEMENTS

Specific recommendations for the use of supplements to treat particular ailments are made throughout. If taking supplements as a general boost, opt for a multi-vitamin or multi-mineral preparation to prevent imbalance. Select reputable brands and consult a medical practitioner over any long-term use (i.e. more then 2–3 months). Do not exceed the recommended dose on the pack. Excessive intake of mineral supplements can be damaging. When taken in excess, the water-soluble vitamins (B and C) are generally excreted, but the fat-soluble group (A, D, E and K) can damage the liver. Do not take fat-soluble vitamin supplements for more than 3–4 weeks without professional advice. Daily recommended doses vary enormously, but in general do not exceed the following:

VITAMIN A – *10,000 IUs daily for children, in pregnancy and for those seeking to become pregnant. 20,000 IUs daily for other adults.*
VITAMIN B^6 – *50 mg daily.*
VITAMIN D – *400 IUs daily.*
VITAMIN E – *600 IUs daily. If taking blood-thinning medication do not take vitamin E except under close medical supervision.*

Abbreviations:
IU International Unit. The potency of vitamins is sometimes measured in IUs. Their equivalent in grams varies according to the vitamin extract used.
mg milligram (one-thousandth of a gram).
µg microgram (one-millionth of a gram).

COUGHS & COLDS

CONVENTIONAL AND HERBAL medicine argue that when stress builds up, opportunist bacteria and viruses move in, causing coughs, colds and flu, although some psychologists reason that these ailments provide the chance to take a much-needed rest from day-to-day responsibilities. Such ailments should not be left untreated, as colds, for example, can easily turn into more serious disorders, or leave lingering coughs and persistent catarrh. Early treatment is the answer.

Chesty coughs

The act of coughing removes irritant particles from the airways. Chesty coughs are loose and produce white, yellow or green phlegm. Coloured phlegm may indicate an infection or bronchitis.

THYME & LUNGWORT SYRUP

This soothing expectorant mixture is made with thyme, a useful antiseptic for the respiratory system, and lungwort leaves, which were once said to resemble diseased lungs, hence the plant's use for chest infections.

~ INGREDIENTS ~
10 g liquorice juice stick (*Glycyrrhiza glabra*)
750 ml water
10 g dried thyme (*Thymus vulgaris*)
10 g dried lungwort leaves (*Pulmonaria officinalis*)
5 g dried cowslip flowers (*Primula veris*)
5 g anise seeds (*Pimpinella anisum*)
500 g runny honey

~ HOW TO MAKE THE SYRUP ~

1 Put the liquorice and water in a pan and heat until the liquorice has dissolved.

2 Mix the herbs and the seeds together and pour on the hot liquorice juice. Infuse for 10 minutes and strain.

3 Return the strained mixture, which should amount to about 500 ml, to the pan and add the honey. Heat the mixture gently until simmering and stir constantly until the honey is dissolved. Allow the mixture to cool, pour into sterilized, dark glass bottles and seal with cork stoppers.

DOSAGE *Take a 5 ml dose up to 6 times a day while symptoms persist.*

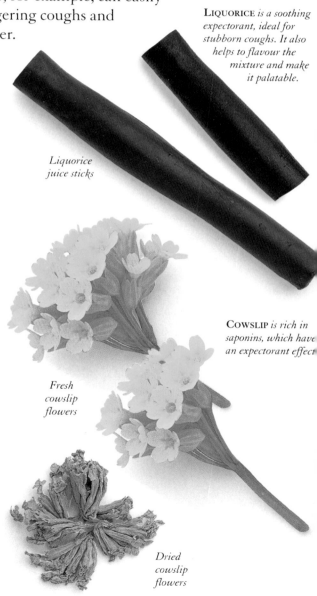

LIQUORICE *is a soothing expectorant, ideal for stubborn coughs. It also helps to flavour the mixture and make it palatable.*

Liquorice juice sticks

COWSLIP *is rich in saponins, which have an expectorant effect*

Fresh cowslip flowers

Dried cowslip flowers

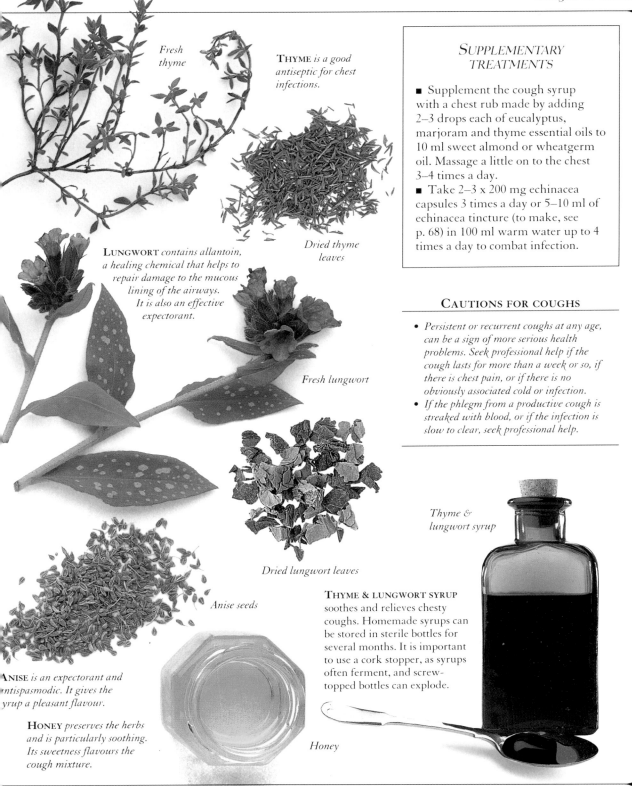

Fresh thyme

THYME *is a good antiseptic for chest infections.*

Dried thyme leaves

LUNGWORT *contains allantoin, a healing chemical that helps to repair damage to the mucous lining of the airways. It is also an effective expectorant.*

Fresh lungwort

Dried lungwort leaves

Anise seeds

ANISE *is an expectorant and antispasmodic. It gives the syrup a pleasant flavour.*

HONEY *preserves the herbs and is particularly soothing. Its sweetness flavours the cough mixture.*

Honey

SUPPLEMENTARY TREATMENTS

■ Supplement the cough syrup with a chest rub made by adding 2–3 drops each of eucalyptus, marjoram and thyme essential oils to 10 ml sweet almond or wheatgerm oil. Massage a little on to the chest 3–4 times a day.

■ Take 2–3 x 200 mg echinacea capsules 3 times a day or 5–10 ml of echinacea tincture (to make, see p. 68) in 100 ml warm water up to 4 times a day to combat infection.

CAUTIONS FOR COUGHS

- *Persistent or recurrent coughs at any age, can be a sign of more serious health problems. Seek professional help if the cough lasts for more than a week or so, if there is chest pain, or if there is no obviously associated cold or infection.*
- *If the phlegm from a productive cough is streaked with blood, or if the infection is slow to clear, seek professional help.*

Thyme & lungwort syrup

THYME & LUNGWORT SYRUP soothes and relieves chesty coughs. Homemade syrups can be stored in sterile bottles for several months. It is important to use a cork stopper, as syrups often ferment, and screw-topped bottles can explode.

Irritant coughs

Irritating, dry or "unproductive" coughs can be debilitating. They are often associated with nervous tension and anxiety, rather than infections, and may respond to soothing cough suppressants.

——— WILD CHERRY & HYSSOP SYRUP ———

Wild cherry is a mild sedative, good for suppressing irritable or racking coughs, or when further coughing is exhausting and unhelpful. It is combined with hyssop, a traditional remedy for stubborn coughs.

~ INGREDIENTS ~
30 g dried wild cherry bark (*Prunus serotina*)
250 ml & 100 ml water
10 g dried hyssop (*Hyssopus officinalis*)
250 g runny honey

~ HOW TO MAKE THE SYRUP ~

1 Soak the cherry bark in 250 ml water overnight. Strain the liquid and reduce slightly by simmering gently for 15 minutes to make a decoction.

2 Meanwhile, make a standard infusion of the hyssop in 100 ml water (see p. 64), strain and add the liquid to the reduced bark decoction.

3 Add the honey and simmer for 5–10 minutes to produce a syrup. Allow the mixture to cool and store in sterilized, dark glass bottles with cork stoppers.

DOSAGE *Take 5 ml up to 4 times a day while symptoms persist.*

Note: see CAUTIONS FOR COUGHS *on p. 85.*

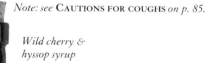

Wild cherry & hyssop syrup

Dried wild cherry bark

Common colds

The common cold is caused by viral infection and is usually characterized by the familiar dry throat and running nose, in some cases progressing to feverishness and persistent coughs.

——— BONESET & ELDERFLOWER TEA ———

Boneset was used in North America for bone-shaking fevers, not for treating fractures as its name may suggest. Elderflower is added to combat catarrh.

~ INGREDIENTS ~
10g dried boneset (*Eupatorium perfoliatum*)
10g dried elderflower (*Sambucus nigra*)
5g dried yarrow (*Achillea millefolium*)
5g dried peppermint (*Mentha piperita*)
500 ml water

~ HOW TO MAKE THE TEA ~

Mix the herbs and place in a teapot and pour on the freshly boiled water. Infuse for 10 minutes and strain into a jug. Cover, and store in a cool place.

DOSAGE *Take a wineglass dose every 3–4 hours as long as symptoms persist. Flavour with honey if desired.*

Supplementary treatments

■ If you feel shivery and chilled, drink a warming decoction of ginger and other spicy herbs to encourage sweating. Try the recipe for Ginger & Cinnamon Tea on p. 108.
■ Take immune stimulants to fight the infection: echinacea – 100 mg tablets up to 4 times daily, or 5 ml of tincture up to 4 times daily; or garlic – one crushed clove 3 times daily, or 2–3 pearls 3 times a day.
■ Eat plenty of fruit and avoid mucus-forming foods, such as dairy products, refined carbohydrates and alcohol.

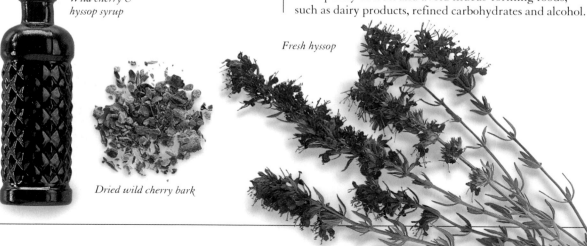

Fresh hyssop

Flu

We often describe a bad cold as flu, but the real thing can also include fever, coughing, head and body pains, nausea and vomiting. It often leaves the sufferer feeling debilitated and depressed for several weeks afterwards.

—— *ELECAMPANE & VERVAIN MIXTURE* ——

Elecampane is an excellent tonic expectorant and restorative, while vervain encourages sweating to help reduce fevers and aids the digestion.

~ INGREDIENTS ~

10g dried elecampane root (*Inula helenium*)
5g dried pleurisy root (*Asclepias tuberosa*)
5g dried vervain (*Verbena officinalis*)
5g dried liquorice root (*Glycyrrhiza glabra*)
5g dried boneset (*Eupatorium perfoliatum*)
500 ml water

~ HOW TO MAKE THE MIXTURE ~

[1] Heat the elecampane and pleurisy root in the water. Simmer gently for 15 minutes to make a decoction. Meanwhile, mix the other herbs in a teapot or lidded jug.

[2] Pour the simmering decoction over the dried herbs. Infuse for 10 minutes and strain. Store in a cool place.

DOSAGE *Take a wineglass dose 3 times a day. Continue taking the mixture for a couple of weeks after the attack as a tonic.*

Supplementary treatments

■ Take the teas described for colds and fevers as necessary.
■ Take 3 x 200 mg echinacea capsules 3 times a day (to make the capsules, see p. 70).
■ Use a compress (to make, see p. 71) soaked in lavender infusion to ease feverish headaches.
■ Drink a standard infusion of St John's wort and lemon balm tea (to make, see p. 64) if depression is a problem.

Fevers

High temperature is part of the body's normal response to infection, and traditional fever management is aimed at helping the body fight infection by either cooling, when need be, with herbs to encourage sweating, or maintaining body temperature with heating remedies.

CAUTION

• *Professional support is needed for high fevers – seek medical help if body temperatures rise over 39°C/102°F.*

—— *CATMINT & VERVAIN TEA* ——

This is a cooling mixture for use when the fever is at the hot, sticky stage. Catmint is a sedative herb that encourages sweating, and vervain is a good digestive stimulant.

~ INGREDIENTS ~

40 g dried catmint (*Nepeta cataria*)
30 g dried vervain (*Verbena officinalis*)
30 g dried boneset (*Eupatorium perfoliatum*)
water

~ HOW TO MAKE THE TEA ~

[1] Mix the herbs and store in a dry, airtight container.

[2] Put 2–3 teaspoonfuls of the mix in a tisane cup or small teapot. Add a cup of freshly boiled water and infuse for 10 minutes. Strain.

DOSAGE *Sip a cup of the mixture as often as possible until body temperature drops.*

Supplementary treatments

■ During the chill stages of a fever drink a warming tea. Try the Ginger & Cinnamon Tea given on p. 108.
■ Take 5–10 ml of echinacea tincture 3 times a day to combat infections (to make, see p. 68).

OVER-THE-COUNTER REMEDIES Coughs & Colds

■ Patent cough and cold remedies are readily available, containing herbs such as astralagus (*Huang Qi*), aniseed, bloodroot, boneset, cowslip, clove, echinacea, ephedra (*Ma Huang*), eucalyptus, fennel, hyssop, ipecacuanha, liquorice, peppermint and sundew.
■ Over-the-counter inhalants can help congestion. They usually contain cajeput, clove, eucalyptus, peppermint and juniper oils, and sometimes added menthol, an active ingredient of peppermint oil.
■ Use elderflower and peppermint teabags together, as a quick option for minor colds. Alternatively, dilute elderflower cordial with hot water and sip.

EARS, NOSE & THROAT

THE MUCOUS MEMBRANES of the nose and throat are the body's first line of defence in keeping dust and toxins out of the system and away from the lungs. Microscopic hair cells constantly beat stray particles out of the way and move them down towards the stomach. These defences have to work overtime in our polluted environment and it is not surprising that sometimes they fail – paving the way for disorders of the nose, throat and ears.

Note: Ears, nose & throat problems can be related to various other disorders. See also coughs & colds pp. 84–6; hayfever p. 100; sinus headaches p. 110.

Sore throats & laryngitis

Sore throats often herald the onset of colds and flu, or they can be a symptom of overworked vocal chords. They may also signal local inflammation and infection as with laryngitis and pharyngitis – inflammations of the vocal chords or nasal cavities.

SAGE & ROSEMARY GARGLE

One of the best combinations for sore throats and laryngitis: both rosemary and sage are aromatic, antiseptic, and rich in potent healing oils. Additional astringents such as lady's mantle can also help reduce inflammation.

~ INGREDIENTS ~

15 g dried, or 45 g fresh red sage leaves
(*Salvia officinalis "purpurea"*)
10 g dried, or 20 g fresh rosemary leaves
(*Rosmarinus officinalis*)
5 g dried lady's mantle leaves (*Alchemilla vulgaris*)
500 ml water

~ HOW TO MAKE THE GARGLE ~

1 Mix the herbs together in a teapot or jug and add freshly boiled water.

2 Infuse for 10 minutes, strain and allow the mixture to cool. Cover and store in a cool place.

DOSAGE *Gargle with a wineglassful at a time every 2–3 hours while symptoms persist. The tea is antiseptic and healing, so swallow the mixture after gargling.*

Supplementary treatments

■ Add 5 ml of echinacea tincture (to make, see p. 68) to each gargle or take separately to combat infections. Take 2–3 garlic pearls daily to support the immune system.
■ Laryngitis and pharyngitis can be helped by steam inhalations: add 2 drops each of sandalwood, frankincense and lavender essential oils to a bowl of boiling water and inhale the steam for 10 minutes (see p. 78). Stay in a warm room for at least 30 minutes afterwards.
■ Add the same oils to 5 ml of sweet almond oil and massage the mixture around the throat.

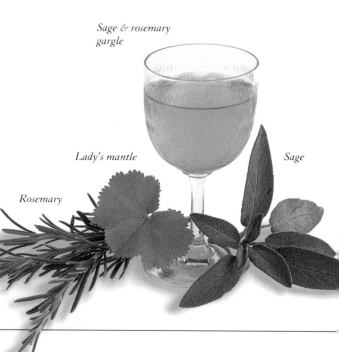

Sage & rosemary gargle

Lady's mantle

Sage

Rosemary

Tonsillitis

The tonsils, at the back of the throat, are a type of lymph gland, part of the body's immune system. Persistent infection can signify weakened immunity or constant underlying physical stress, such as food intolerance or exhaustion. Cutting out potential irritant foods, such as milk or wheat, may help – so can a good relaxing holiday.

CLEAVERS & SAGE TINCTURE

Cleavers is cleansing and healing for the lymphatic system. In this remedy it is combined with sage, an antiseptic, and other antibacterials and immune stimulants, to help combat tonsillitis.

~ INGREDIENTS ~
50 ml cleavers tincture (*Galium aparine*)
15 ml sage tincture (*Salvia officinalis*)
25 ml echinacea tincture (*Echinacea angustifolia*)
10 ml goldenseal tincture (*Hydrastis canadensis*)

~ HOW TO MAKE THE TINCTURE ~
1 To make the individual tinctures, see p. 68.

2 Combine all the tinctures in a sterilized dark glass bottle and mix well.

DOSAGE *Take 10 ml of the mixture in half a tumbler of hot water 3 times a day during the acute stage, adding a little honey if desired. Reduce to 5 ml in hot water 3 times a day, as symptoms ease.*

CAUTIONS
• *Abscesses on the tonsils (quinsy) need professional help.*
• *Seek help if there is fever, especially in children.*

Supplementary treatments
■ Use the gargle on p. 88 for sore throats, substituting thyme leaves for rosemary, as they are more antiseptic.
■ Strengthen the immune system by taking either 1 g vitamin C, 2–3 garlic pearls or 2–3 x 200 mg *Huang Qi* capsules daily for a few weeks to help prevent attacks recurring.
■ Drink a soothing infusion daily made with 10 g each of dried ground ivy, pot marigold petals and chamomile flowers (to make, see p. 64).
■ Add 5 drops each of thyme and marjoram essential oils and a single drop of rose oil to 25 ml of sweet almond oil and massage into the neck area. Use the same mix of oils in a steam inhalation (to make, see p. 78).

Mouth ulcers

Painful ulcers in the mouth – known as aphthae – are often related to opportunist fungal or bacterial infections gaining a hold when sufferers are exhausted and run down. Sometimes ulcers are associated with excessive sugar consumption, which fuels fungal growths. They can also be linked to stomach upsets.

MYRRH & ROSEMARY MOUTHWASH

Myrrh is extremely antimicrobial. It is one of the less pleasant-tasting herbs, however, and rosemary infusion is added to help disguise the flavour.

~ INGREDIENTS ~
15 ml myrrh tincture or 5 drops myrrh oil (*Commiphora molmol*)
30 g dried rosemary (*Rosmarinus officinalis*)
500 ml water

~ HOW TO MAKE THE MOUTHWASH ~
1 To make the tincture, see p. 68.

2 Put the rosemary in a jug or teapot and add freshly boiled water. Infuse for 10 minutes and strain.

3 Add the myrrh tincture or myrrh oil to the rosemary infusion and stir well. Cover and store in a cool place.

DOSAGE *Use a wineglass of the mixture as a mouthwash every 4 hours until symptoms ease.*

Supplementary treatments
■ Chew bilberries after the mouthwash to help disguise the flavour and promote healing.
■ Apply a drop of clove oil directly to the mouth ulcer – this will probably sting, but it can be very effective.
■ Take 2 x 200 mg echinacea capsules 3 times a day to combat infection.
■ Persistent fungal infections may be the cause of mouth ulcers. Avoid sugary food and dairy products, eat plenty of garlic and take marigold infusion (to make, see p. 64) as a daily tea.
■ Take professional advice if mouth ulcers are persistent or severe as they can be related to food intolerance. In particular, they commonly indicate sensitivity to gluten. They may also be a sign of iron deficiency, or of vitamins B[12] or B[6], or of folic acid.

Catarrh

The protective membranes lining the nasal passages produce mucus as a form of protection in response to infections or irritants. Excess mucus – catarrh – often follows a common cold, and is also caused by allergens, such as pollen and house dust.

——— SANDALWOOD & PINE INHALANT———

Steam inhalants are one of the most effective ways of treating upper respiratory tract problems. These oils are astringent, antiseptic and soothing.

~ INGREDIENTS ~
15 drops sandalwood oil (*Santalum album*)
15 drops pine oil (*Pinus sylvestris*)
10 drops lavender oil (*Lavandula angustifolia*)
5 drops peppermint oil (*Mentha piperita*)
45 ml compound tincture of benzoin
– friar's balsam (*Styrax benzoin*)

~ HOW TO USE THE INHALANT ~

1 Mix the ingredients in a 50 ml sterilized, dark glass bottle and shake well.

2 Fill a basin with boiling water. Add a teaspoon of the mix to the water. Lean over the water and cover the head and basin with a towel. Inhale the steam for 10 minutes. Repeat twice a day while catarrh persists.

Note: Stay in a warm room for at least 30 minutes afterwards.

Supplementary treatments
■ Mix 30 ml each of eyebright, ribwort plantain and echinacea tinctures with 10 ml of goldenseal tincture (to make, see p. 68). Sip a 5 ml dose diluted in warm water 3 times a day.
■ Take 2 x 200 mg garlic capsules 3 times a day.

Sinusitis

The sinuses are cavities in the skull. They can be prone to inflammation and overproduction of mucus, leading to headaches, gum pains and watery eyes. Learning to relax and manage stress has a marked effect on sinusitis, and the condition often responds to the action of warming herbs.

— MAGNOLIA & ELDERFLOWER TINCTURE —

Magnolia is an excellent anti-inflammatory for the mucous membranes, and elderflower is a traditional remedy for catarrh and phlegm.

~ INGREDIENTS ~
25 ml magnolia flower tincture
(*Xin Yi Hua – Magnolia liliflora*)
25 ml elderflower tincture (*Sambucus nigra*)
15 ml ground ivy tincture (*Glechoma hederacea*)
15 ml echinacea tincture (*Echinacea angustifolia*)
10 ml bayberry tincture (*Myrica cerifera*)
5 ml ginger tincture (*Zingiber officinalis*)
5 ml peppermint tincture (*Mentha piperita*)

~ HOW TO MAKE THE TINCTURE ~

To make the individual tinctures, see p. 68. Combine them in a 100 ml sterilized, dark glass bottle and shake well.

DOSAGE *Take 5 ml in half a tumbler of warm water 3 times a day before meals while symptoms persist.*

Supplementary treatments
■ Make a cream (see p. 76) by adding 10 ml bayberry tincture and 5 ml elderflower tincture (to make, see p. 68) to 50 ml melted emulsifying ointment (available over the counter). Apply the cream to the sinus areas 2 or 3 times a day, massaging gently.
■ Add 5 drops of sandalwood oil to a saucer of water on the bedside table to relieve symptoms at night.
■ Take 2 x 200 mg capsules of dried, powdered garlic 3 times a day and take extra vitamin C. A 24- or 48-hour fruit fast may help. (The weak or elderly should take professional advice before fasting.)
■ See p. 110 for advice on treating sinus headaches.

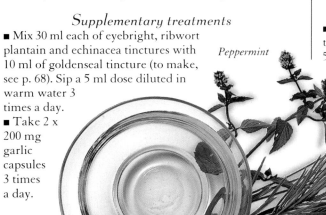

Peppermint

Lavender

Sandalwood & pine inhalant

Pine

Sandalwood

Earache

Earache may be caused by local acute infection, but can also be related to sinus problems, catarrh, toothache or mumps. Identifying the cause is important. Recurring ear infections, especially in children, can be associated with food intolerance (see p. 101).

CAUTIONS

- *Seek professional help if pain is severe, especially in children. Get help: if there is pain in the mastoid bone (behind the ear); if there is a discharge from the ear; or if the condition persists.*
- *Do not put anything into the ear if the eardrum is perforated; seek medical advice if unsure.*

— MULLEIN & PASQUE FLOWER EARDROPS —

Pasque flower is a good sedative and analgesic that seems to have a specific affinity with the ears, while mullein is a herb with soothing properties that helps repair damaged tissues.

~ INGREDIENTS ~

20 drops pasque flower tincture (*Anemone vulgaris*)
24 ml infused mullein oil (*Verbascum thapsus*)
20 drops goldenseal tincture (*Hydrastis canadensis*)

~ HOW TO MAKE THE EARDROPS ~

To make the tinctures and infused oil see pp. 68 and 72. Mix the ingredients in a sterilized dropper bottle. Shake.

APPLICATION *Using the dropper, put 2 drops into the ear and cover with a cottonwool plug. Repeat 3 times a day.*

Supplementary treatments

■ Massage the mastoid bone (behind the ear), in front of the ear and at the back of the neck with a mix of 2 ml each of lavender and tea tree oil in 20 ml of sweet almond oil to reduce the risk of infection spreading.
■ Take 5 ml echinacea tincture (see p. 68) or 2–3 garlic pearls 3 times daily and a zinc and vitamin C supplement.
■ Avoid mucus-forming foods such as dairy products.

Chronic ear infection

Inflammation of the middle ear (*otitis media*) is common at all ages. When it causes fluid to collect it can lead to deafness and this condition (glue ear) is most common in children. In addition to progressive hearing loss, it is characterized by earache and copious sticky secretions. Some researchers have associated it with allergy to cow's milk. Orthodox treatment usually involves inserting grommets in the eardrum to relieve the build-up of fluid.

—— GOLDEN ROD & GINKGO MIXTURE ——

Golden rod is a good anticatarrhal that can be helpful in ear conditions, while both ginkgo and pasque flower have an affinity with ear problems, helping to focus healing mixtures on the ear. The dose given here is suitable for children aged 4–6, the most frequent sufferers. See p. 128 for general advice on children's dosage.

~ INGREDIENTS ~

40 ml golden rod tincture (*Solidago virgaurea*)
25 ml ginkgo tincture (*Ginkgo biloba*)
15 ml ribwort plantain tincture (*Plantago lanceolata*)
10 ml St John's wort tincture (*Hypericum perforatum*)
10 ml pasque flower tincture (*Anemone vulgaris*)

~ HOW TO MAKE THE MIXTURE ~

To make the individual tinctures, see p. 68. Combine them in a 100 ml sterilized, dark glass bottle and shake well.

DOSAGE *Take 20 drops in a glass of fruit juice 3 times a day.*

Supplementary treatments

■ Take a 200 mg goldenseal capsule daily. Alternatively, add 5 ml of goldenseal tincture to the main remedy and use a strongly flavoured juice, such as blackcurrant, to dilute the mixture, as goldenseal has a very bitter taste.
■ Replace cow's milk in the diet with soya products and reduce sugar intake as much as possible.

OVER-THE-COUNTER REMEDIES *Ears, Nose & Throat*

■ For catarrhal problems, look out for capsules or tablets combining any of the following astringent, antiseptic, soothing herbs: agrimony, bayberry bark, cloves, elderflower, ephedra (*Ma Huang*), eucalyptus, eyebright, golden rod, goldenseal, magnolia flowers, marshmallow, peppermint, white horehound, wild indigo and yarrow.

■ Look for ready-mixed inhalants, such as those based on friar's balsam.
■ Try herbal nasal sprays that combine eucalyptus and peppermint oils.
■ Use herbal teabags containing elderflower, pot marigold, or peppermint to supplement other therapeutic approaches.

EYE COMPLAINTS

THE EYES ARE in constant use transmitting images, a task made much harder by having to cope with computer screens, the dust and grit of city streets, and sunlight that is becoming progressively brighter, due to ozone depletion. Regular exercises, such as alternately focusing on near and distant objects, can help hardworking eyes. Splashing them with cold water each morning can also help to keep them working well. Herbal remedies are very useful for soothing the symptoms of many common eye complaints.

GENERAL CAUTION
• *Eye infections can be very contagious – avoid sharing face towels or face flannels.*

Styes

A stye is an inflammation of the glands found at the base of the eyelashes. It is caused by a bacterial infection and is generally a sign that the sufferer is run down. Rest, relaxation and a good diet are just as important as topical treatments.

─── *MARIGOLD COMPRESS* ───

Astringent and antiseptic, marigold is an excellent remedy for local skin infections and inflammations.

~ INGREDIENTS ~
25 g dried pot marigold petals (*Calendula officinalis*)
500 ml water

~ HOW TO MAKE THE COMPRESS ~

1 Pour freshly boiled water on to the pot marigold petals. Infuse for 10 minutes and strain.

2 As soon as the infusion is cool enough to handle, soak a small square of muslin or other cloth in it.

APPLICATION *Wring out the cloth and apply it to the stye, holding it to the affected area until the compress cools. Repeat with a fresh compress at frequent intervals during the day, reheating the infusion as necessary, until the infection subsides. Make a fresh infusion daily.*

Supplementary treatments
■ Boost the immune system with either 2–3 garlic pearls 3 times a day or 2 x 200 mg echinacea capsules 3 times a day.
■ Drink an infusion 2 or 3 times daily made from equal parts of cleavers, *Ju Hua* (dried Chinese chrysanthemum flowers), fumitory and burdock leaf. (To make, see p. 64.)

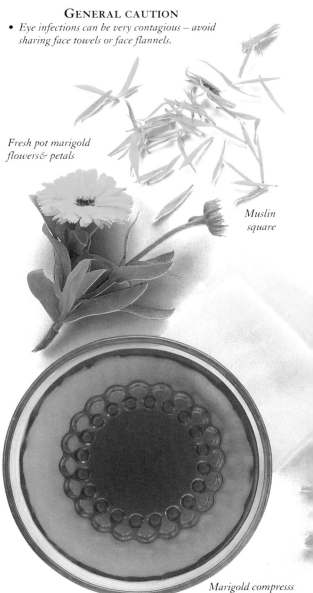

Fresh pot marigold flowers & petals

Muslin square

Marigold compress

Conjunctivitis & blepharitis

Conjunctivitis, commonly known as "red eye", is an inflammation of the mucous membrane covering the eyeball. Blepharitis is inflammation of the eyelid. Both are usually caused by infection, although conjunctivitis can also be associated with dusty, polluted air, or a drying of the eye's normal secretions in old age.

—— EYEBRIGHT & MARIGOLD EYEBATH ——

Eyebright, as its name suggests, is a herb traditionally used to treat eye infections. It is a tiny, semi-parasitic plant found in grass meadows but rarely grown in herb gardens.

~ INGREDIENTS ~
15 g dried eyebright (*Euphrasia officinalis*)
10 g dried pot marigold petals (*Calendula officinalis*)
500 ml water

~ HOW TO MAKE THE EYEBATH ~
1 Mix the herbs and water together and heat in a pan.

2 Simmer for 5–10 minutes to sterilize the herbs. Strain, and allow to cool completely. Store in a sterilized bottle.

APPLICATION *Pour a little into a sterilized eyebath and bathe the eye thoroughly. If both eyes are affected, sterilize the eyebath again and pour a fresh amount of the mixture into the eyebath, before bathing the other eye. Repeat frequently in acute cases. Make a fresh mixture each day. Note: see p. 62 for advice on sterilizing.*

CAUTION
• *Seek professional help if the infection does not resolve within a day or so, or if there is decreased vision or pain in the eye.*

Supplementary treatments
■ Apply cold, used teabags of Indian, Chinese or fennel tea to the eyes as poultices, and relax for 15 minutes.
■ To combat infection, drink a standard infusion of eyebright 3 times a day (to make, see p. 64), and take 2–3 garlic pearls 3 times a day or 2 x 200 mg echinacea capsules 3 times a day.

Tired eyes & eye strain

Stress, long working hours and pollution all combine to make eye strain a common problem. The simple answer is to take regular breaks from computer screens, avoid working all day in artificial light, frequently focus on distant objects for a few seconds as a break from close work, or close the eyes and press very gently on the eyelids with the palms.

—— JU HUA & WOOD BETONY TEA ——

In Chinese medicine the eyes are associated with the liver, and herbs such as Ju Hua and wood betony, which clean and stimulate that organ, can also help to revive the eyes.

~ INGREDIENTS ~
25 g *Ju Hua* (dried, prepared Chinese chrysanthemum flowers – *Chrysanthemum morifolium*)
20 g dried wood betony (*Stachys betonica*)
10 g dried *gotu kola* (*Centella asiatica*)
5 g dried peppermint (*Mentha piperita*)
water

~ HOW TO MAKE THE TEA ~
1 Mix the herbs and store in a dark, airtight container.

2 Put 2–3 teaspoons of the mix in a tisane cup or small teapot. Add a cup of freshly boiled water and infuse for 10 minutes. Strain.

DOSAGE *Take a break from work and drink a cup when the eyes feel tired.*

Supplementary treatments
■ Place slices of fresh cucumber on each closed eye and relax for 10–15 minutes.
■ Take vitamin C and vitamin A supplements, or eat a few carrots each day.
■ Bathe the eyes with Eyebright & Marigold Eyebath (left) or with 5 drops of self-heal tincture (to make, see p. 68) in an eyebath of warm water.

Fresh pot marigold

OVER-THE-COUNTER REMEDIES *Eye Complaints*

■ Apply a tiny dab of ready-made calendula cream directly to styes.
■ Use shop-bought elderflower, fennel, pot marigold or raspberry leaf teabags to make an infusion. Allow to cool and then apply them to inflamed and tired eyes as a cold poultice to relieve symptoms.

SKIN & HAIR PROBLEMS

THE SKIN FORMS A remarkable defensive barrier against the outside world. It harbours a thriving community of bacteria to ward off unfriendly micro-organisms and contains millions of sensory nerve endings. Its efficiency is a good guide to our general health and well-being, and herbal remedies for skin complaints usually focus on internal medication to restore a healthy balance in the body.

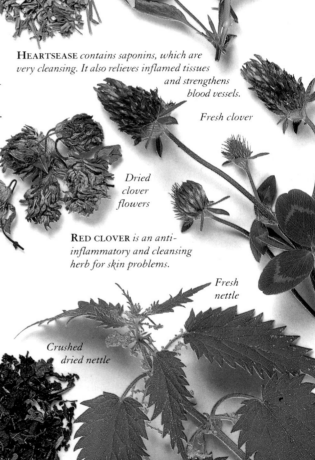

Dried heartsease aerial parts

Fresh heartsease

HEARTSEASE *contains saponins, which are very cleansing. It also relieves inflamed tissues and strengthens blood vessels.*

Fresh clover

Dried clover flowers

RED CLOVER *is an anti-inflammatory and cleansing herb for skin problems.*

Eczema

Irritant skin inflammation may be due to allergy – from food (see p. 101) or contact with particular chemicals – and can often become worse with stress. Calming remedies can help to reduce attacks, and cleansing herbs remove toxins from the system.

—— HEARTSEASE & RED CLOVER TEA ——

Heartsease is a good cleansing and anti-inflammatory herb that also acts as a gentle circulatory stimulant. Red clover also helps clear toxins from the system and has a diuretic action.

~ INGREDIENTS ~
20 g dried heartsease (*Viola tricolor*)
20 g dried red clover flowers (*Trifolium pratense*)
20 g dried stinging nettle (*Urtica dioica*)
20 g dried burdock (*Arctium lappa*)
10 g dried fumitory (*Fumaria officinalis*)
10 g dried skullcap (*Scutellaria lateriflora*)
500 ml water

~ HOW TO MAKE THE TEA ~

1 Mix the herbs and store in an airtight jar. Spoon 25 g of the mixture into a teapot.

2 Pour 500 ml of freshly boiled water on to the mixture. Infuse for 10 minutes and strain. Cover and store the surplus in a cool place.

DOSAGE *Take a wineglass dose 3 times a day before meals. (See p. 83 for advice on length of treatment.)*

Fresh nettle

Crushed dried nettle

STINGING NETTLE *is rich in vitamins and minerals and stimulates the circulation.*

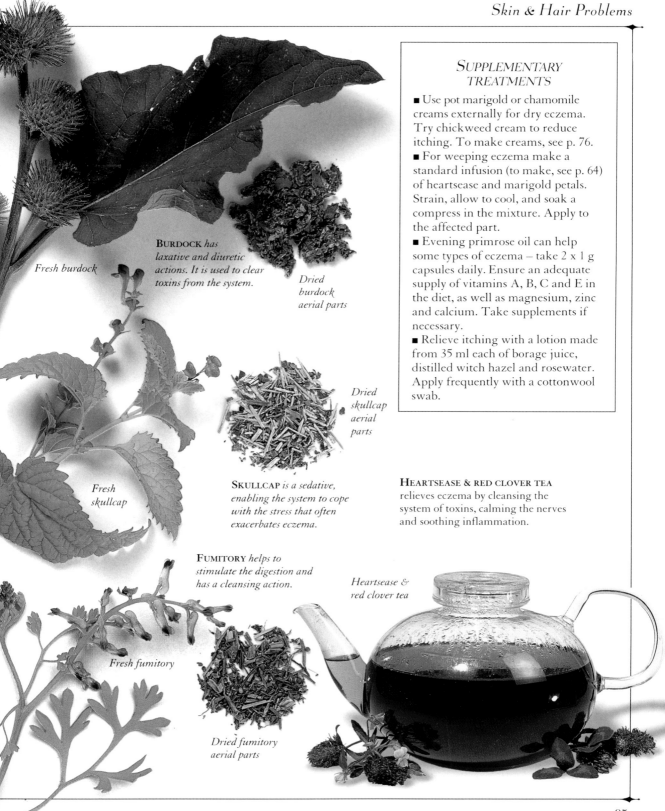

Fresh burdock

BURDOCK *has laxative and diuretic actions. It is used to clear toxins from the system.*

Dried burdock aerial parts

SUPPLEMENTARY TREATMENTS

■ Use pot marigold or chamomile creams externally for dry eczema. Try chickweed cream to reduce itching. To make creams, see p. 76.
■ For weeping eczema make a standard infusion (to make, see p. 64) of heartsease and marigold petals. Strain, allow to cool, and soak a compress in the mixture. Apply to the affected part.
■ Evening primrose oil can help some types of eczema – take 2 x 1 g capsules daily. Ensure an adequate supply of vitamins A, B, C and E in the diet, as well as magnesium, zinc and calcium. Take supplements if necessary.
■ Relieve itching with a lotion made from 35 ml each of borage juice, distilled witch hazel and rosewater. Apply frequently with a cottonwool swab.

Dried skullcap aerial parts

Fresh skullcap

SKULLCAP *is a sedative, enabling the system to cope with the stress that often exacerbates eczema.*

HEARTSEASE & RED CLOVER TEA relieves eczema by cleansing the system of toxins, calming the nerves and soothing inflammation.

FUMITORY *helps to stimulate the digestion and has a cleansing action.*

Heartsease & red clover tea

Fresh fumitory

Dried fumitory aerial parts

Psoriasis

Psoriasis involves over-production of certain skin cells, which causes patches of silvery scaling usually found on the knees, elbows or scalp. It is quite common in the West and in rare cases it can become very severe, affecting large parts of the body and may be associated with chronic rheumatic disorders.

—————— FIGWORT TEA ——————

Psoriasis is an ailment that seems to come and go, and is often helped by sunshine and sea bathing. Cleansing, anti-inflammatory herbs, such as figwort and red clover can also help.

~ INGREDIENTS ~

10 g fresh burdock root (*Arctium lappa*)
5 g fresh yellow dock root (*Rumex crispus*)
15 g fresh figwort (*Scrophularia nodosa*)
10 g fresh red clover flowers (*Trifolium pratense*)
750 ml water

~ HOW TO MAKE THE TEA ~

1 Mix the burdock and yellow dock together in a pan and add the water. Bring to the boil and simmer for 15 minutes, to make a decoction.

2 Put the figwort and red clover flowers together in a teapot or jug. Pour the burdock and yellow dock decoction over these herbs and infuse for 10 minutes. Strain. Store in a covered jug.

DOSAGE *Take a wineglass dose 3 times a day. See p. 83 for advice on how long to take. Flavour with honey or lemon juice as required.*

Supplementary treatments

■ Cleavers cream (to make, see p. 76) can be useful for treating small patches or the early stages of psoriasis. Apply a little 2 or 3 times a day to affected areas.
■ If the scalp is affected, make a hair rinse using 10 ml of rosemary tincture (to make, see p. 68) and 10 drops of cade oil in 500 ml of warm water. Apply after shampooing as a final rinse.
■ Psoriasis often seems to go with a tense, insular personality. Bach Flower Remedies such as crab apple, agrimony, willow or water violet can sometimes help.
■ Avoid alcohol and herbs such as yarrow, cinnamon twigs and linden flowers, as these increase peripheral circulation and so stimulate the skin.
■ Take 1 g vitamin C and 1–2 g kelp daily. Take zinc and vitamin A tablets also (follow the instructions on the pack).

Urticaria (hives)

Urticaria and hives are names for a rash of red, itchy lumps and blisters on the skin. They can be caused by contact with irritant allergens, such as those found in plants like stinging nettles, hops, runner beans or borage. Chemicals such as salicylates, found in aspirin and in many foods, can have a similar effect, causing rashes that occur around the mouth.

—————— AGRIMONY & CHAMOMILE TEA ——————

Persistent urticaria is generally related to food allergies. This soothing infusion contains agrimony, a useful herb for calming gut irritations, and chamomile, which has anti-allergenic properties.

~ INGREDIENTS ~

10 g dried agrimony (*Agrimonia eupatoria*)
10 g dried chamomile flowers (*Matricaria recutita*)
5 g dried stinging nettles (*Urtica dioica*)
5 g dried heartsease (*Viola tricolor*)
500 ml water

~ HOW TO MAKE THE TEA ~

Mix the herbs and put in a teapot. Add the freshly boiled water. Infuse for 5 minutes and strain into a jug. Cover and store in a cool place.

DOSAGE *Take a wineglass dose 3 times a day until the rash subsides.*

Supplementary treatments

■ Rub the area with sliced onion or crushed cabbage leaves.
■ Use chamomile cream (available over the counter – to make, see p. 76) on affected areas several times a day.
■ If stress is a contributory factor, drink an infusion of skullcap (to make, see p. 64) 3 times a day.

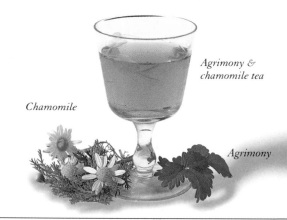

Agrimony & chamomile tea

Chamomile

Agrimony

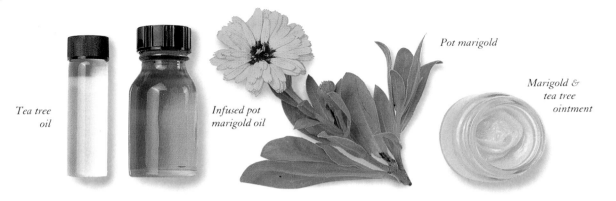

Tea tree oil

Infused pot marigold oil

Pot marigold

Marigold & tea tree ointment

Ringworm & athlete's foot

Skin infections, like ringworm and athlete's foot, are often caused by common fungi, which attack when the immune system is weakened by stress or exhaustion. Fungi thrive in damp, confined conditions, for example between poorly washed or dried toes.

—— MARIGOLD & TEA TREE OINTMENT ——

Both pot marigold and tea tree are extremely antifungal. Using an ointment helps to keep the affected areas dry, which discourages the fungi. Combining the two oils for use as a lotion is a convenient alternative.

~ INGREDIENTS ~
25 ml infused pot marigold oil (*Calendula officinalis*)
8 g beeswax
8 g anhydrous lanolin
5 ml tea tree oil (*Melaleuca alternifolia*)

~ HOW TO MAKE THE OINTMENT ~

1 To make the infused pot marigold oil, see p. 73.

2 Melt the beeswax and anhydrous lanolin in a double saucepan. Warm the pot marigold oil slightly in a second double saucepan.

3 Combine the two mixtures and remove from the heat, stirring well.

4 When the mixture has started to cool significantly, but before it sets, add the tea tree oil. Stir. Pour into a sterilized dark glass jar and allow the mixture to set.

APPLICATION *Rub gently on affected areas several times a day while symptoms persist.*

Boils & carbuncles

Boils occur when a hair follicle becomes inflamed and infected by bacteria. A cluster of boils is known as a carbuncle. Recurrent boils indicate weakened resistance to disease through stress, exhaustion or an underlying deep-seated infection, such as a dental abscess. Improving diet and lifestyle can help.

—— SLIPPERY ELM POULTICE ——

Hot poultices are very effective at drawing the core from boils. Slippery elm is ideal for this, with a few drops of eucalyptus oil added as an antiseptic.

~ INGREDIENTS ~
25 g powdered slippery elm (*Ulmus fulva*)
3 drops eucalyptus oil (*Eucalyptus globulus*)
water

~ HOW TO APPLY THE POULTICE ~

1 Add a little boiling water to the slippery elm powder to form a paste.

2 Mix in the eucalyptus oil.

3 Spread the hot mixture on the boil or carbuncle and cover with gauze. Reapply the hot mixture repeatedly each time the poultice cools, until the pus is discharged.

Supplementary treatments
■ To improve resistance to infection, take 2–3 garlic pearls or 5 ml of echinacea tincture (to make, see p. 68) 3 times a day.
■ Drink an infusion made from equal parts of dried honeysuckle flowers, figwort leaves and thyme (to make, see p. 64) to help combat infection and cleanse the system.

Acne

Acne occurs most commonly in teenagers, and is characterized by blackheads, pustules and cysts, caused by inflamed sebaceous glands in the skin. Poor diet is often a contributing factor. Although acne generally clears by the time sufferers reach their early 20s, it can persist into middle age, possibly as a result of hormonal imbalance.

—— LAVENDER & YARROW FACIAL ——

In this two-part treatment, steam is used to open the pores and then a lotion is applied to cleanse the skin. The antiseptic and anti-inflammatory herbs that are added to the steam help to combat the symptoms of acne.

~ INGREDIENTS ~

5 drops tea tree oil (*Melaleuca alternifolia*)
25 ml rosewater (*Rosa damascena*)
25 ml distilled witch hazel (*Hamamelis virginiana*)
10 g dried lavender flowers (*Lavandula angustifolia*)
10 g dried yarrow flowers (*Achillea millefolium*)
10 g dried elderflowers (*Sambucus nigra*)
water

~ HOW TO MAKE THE FACIAL ~

1 Combine the tea tree oil with the rosewater and witch hazel to make an astringent lotion.

2 Mix the lavender, yarrow and elderflowers in a basin and pour boiling water over the mixture.

APPLICATION *Drape a towel over the head and basin and steam the face for 5–10 minutes, before cleansing with the lotion. Repeat once a day.*

Supplementary treatments

■ Take supplements of evening primrose oil, vitamin B-complex, vitamin C and zinc (follow the instructions on the pack), and eat plenty of fresh vegetables and fruit.
■ Blend 3 cabbage leaves with 50 ml distilled witch hazel in a food processor and use as a lotion twice a day.

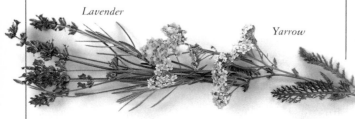

Lavender

Yarrow

Dandruff

Small flakes of dead skin on the scalp, known as dandruff, can be a sign of psoriasis, although they are more commonly associated with seborrhoeic dermatitis or yeast infection.

—— ROSEMARY & NETTLE SHAMPOO ——

Rosemary is a stimulating, warming herb that is a traditional hair rinse, helping to keep hair shiny and healthy. Stinging nettle root is a favourite hair conditioner in many parts of Europe.

~ INGREDIENTS ~

25 g fresh rosemary leaves (*Rosmarinus officinalis*)
10 g fresh, well-washed, stinging nettle root
(*Urtica dioica*)
5 drops tea tree oil (*Melaleuca alternifolia*)
20 g soft soap
100 ml methylated alcohol
350 ml water

~ HOW TO MAKE THE SHAMPOO ~

1 Mix the herbs, oil, soap and alcohol in a 500 ml jar or wide-necked bottle. Add the water and shake well.

2 Leave to infuse for 2 weeks, shaking at regular intervals. Strain into a clean bottle.

APPLICATION *Use as a shampoo 2 or 3 times a week until the dandruff disappears.*

Alopecia

As men age, gradual hair loss (baldness) often occurs. It tends to be hereditary and non-reversible. Where hair loss is sudden or patchy, as in alopecia, stress or vitamin deficiency may be to blame. It is found most commonly in teenagers and young adults.

Treatments

■ Apply arnica cream to the bald patches caused by alopecia (but do not use on broken skin).
■ Rinse the hair with standard infusions (to make, see p. 64) of rosemary, sage or stinging nettle.
■ Take vitamin B and evening primrose oil supplements.
■ If stress is a factor, drink an infusion of equal amounts of skullcap and wood betony (to make, see p. 64).

Cold sores

Once infected with the *Herpes simplex* virus, sufferers develop cold sores whenever the immune system is under stress. The sores usually occur in the same place, and are heralded by a pricking sensation in the skin. The best approach is to avoid recurrence by staying fit and healthy.

───── *TEA TREE & LAVENDER OIL* ─────

Research has shown that a few herbs display specific antiviral properties and can be used topically to treat infections caused by viruses like Herpes simplex. *Use this lotion at the first suggestion of a cold sore.*

~ INGREDIENTS ~
8 ml tea tree oil (*Melaleuca alternifolia*)
5 ml lavender oil (*Lavandula angustifolia*)
12 ml sweet almond oil

~ HOW TO MAKE THE OIL ~
Combine the oils in a sterilized 25 ml dropper bottle and shake well.

APPLICATION *Dab 1–2 drops of the oil on the affected area. Repeat every 2 hours.*

Warts & verrucae

Caused by a viral infection, warts and verrucae can be very contagious. Numerous folk remedies exist – one of the simplest is to apply a few drops of fresh dandelion or greater celandine sap daily.

───── *THUJA & TEA TREE LOTION* ─────

Thuja is a traditional remedy for treating warts and tea tree has powerful antiseptic and antifungal properties.

~ INGREDIENTS ~
15 ml thuja tincture (*Thuja occidentalis*)
10 ml tea tree oil (*Melaleuca alternifolia*)

~ HOW TO MAKE THE LOTION ~
To make the tincture, see p. 68. Combine the tincture and the oil in a sterilized 25 ml dropper bottle. Shake vigorously to form an emulsion.

APPLICATION *Dab 1–2 drops of the mix on the affected area. Repeat up to 4 times a day, shaking the bottle thoroughly before use.*

Impetigo

Impetigo is a common bacterial infection, usually affecting the mouth, nose and ears and producing a crusted discharge. It is highly contagious and is common in children. Topical use of antibiotics is often needed, but the following supplementary measures can help relieve the problem.

Treatments
■ Take 2 x 200 mg garlic capsules or 5 ml echinacea tincture (to make, see p. 68) 3 times a day.
■ Combine 20 ml echinacea tincture, 30 ml pot marigold tincture (to make, see p. 68) and 50 ml witch hazel, and use as a lotion, bathing the affected area 3 or 4 times a day.

Scabies

Scabies are tiny mites that burrow into the skin. They are highly contagious and irritant, and it is important to take professional advice. The following steps will help to combat the condition.

Treatments
■ Add 250 ml of a standard infusion of tansy (to make, see p. 64) to a hot bath at night. Combine 10 ml of tea tree oil and 90 ml of distilled witch hazel and use as a lotion after bathing. Repeat for 3 nights in a row.
■ Boil all clothing and bed linen and leave at least 3 weeks before using, as scabies' eggs can survive for 2 weeks.

CAUTIONS FOR IMPETIGO & SCABIES
• *Scabies and impetigo are extremely contagious: do not share towels or face cloths with the rest of the household.*

OVER-THE-COUNTER REMEDIES
Skin & Hair Problems

■ Many commercially available skin and hair beauty treatments contain herbal products. Usually the amount of herbal extract is far too small to be therapeutic, so look instead for more obviously medicinal products. Pot marigold cream is readily available – usually sold as calendula. Chickweed and chamomile creams and ointments are also produced commercially.
■ Cleansing herbs, such as burdock, cleavers, dandelion, figwort, fumitory and yellow dock are used in patent remedies for skin or hair problems. It is important to follow the instructions given, as most are digestive stimulants and excess intake can lead to diarrhoea.
■ Soap bark is an excellent cleanser for dandruff.

ALLERGIES

IN OUR POLLUTED WORLD allergic reactions are all too common. The body has to cope with a growing variety of alien chemicals, due to ever-increasing levels of irritant exhaust fumes, as well as new strains of agricultural crops, such as oil-seed rape, and food that is often contaminated with pesticides and artificial growth stimulants. In response, the immune system treats the "unknowns" as dangerous, and inflammations and excessive mucus can result as part of the body's defence mechanisms.

Hayfever & allergic rhinitis

Usually triggered by seasonal grass or tree pollens, the familiar sneezing, sore eyes and running nose characteristic of hayfever can also be caused by a reaction to house dust, car fumes or animal hairs, when it is generally referred to as allergic rhinitis. Severe cases can lead to asthma-like symptoms.

— *ELDERFLOWER & DANDELION TINCTURE* —

Hayfever is often best treated in early spring, before the pollen arrives. This tincture, containing elderflower to strengthen the mucous membranes and dandelion to cleanse the liver, will help the system cope with future allergens and so reduce symptoms. This remedy is also suitable for allergic rhinitis.

~ INGREDIENTS ~
25 ml elderflower tincture (*Sambucus nigra*)
20 ml dandelion root tincture (*Taraxacum officinale*)
20 ml vervain tincture (*Verbena officinalis*)
15 ml Siberian ginseng tincture
(*Eleutherococcus senticosus*)
15 ml white horehound tincture (*Marrubium vulgare*)
5 ml liquorice tincture (*Glycyrrhiza glabra*)

~ HOW TO MAKE THE TINCTURE ~

To make the individual tinctures, see p. 68. Mix the tinctures together in a 100 ml sterilized, dark glass bottle.

DOSAGE *Take 5 ml in 100 ml of warm water 3 times a day before meals. For hayfever, take for up to 4 weeks during the spring.*

Supplementary treatments
■ To relieve hayfever symptoms, bathe the eyes with Marigold & Eyebright Eyebath (see p. 93), and take 2 x 200 mg eyebright capsules up to 3 times a day.

Asthma

Allergic asthma is often linked with allergic eczema and starts in childhood. It is caused by a tightening of the small bronchial tubes and production of thick sticky mucus, which makes breathing difficult with a characteristic wheeze.

—— *SUNDEW & HYSSOP MIXTURE* ——

Use of many of the most effective herbs for asthma is restricted to professional practitioners and licensed over-the-counter products. Sundew, an antispasmodic and relaxing expectorant, is one of the best generally available alternatives.

~ INGREDIENTS ~
10 ml sundew fluid extract (*Drosera rotundifolia*)
25 ml hyssop tincture (*Hyssopus officinalis*)
20 ml elecampane tincture (*Inula helenium*)
20 ml thyme tincture (*Thymus vulgaris*)
20 ml chamomile tincture (*Matricaria recutita*)
5 ml liquorice fluid extract (*Glycyrrhiza glabra*)

~ HOW TO MAKE THE MIXTURE ~

To make the individual tinctures, see p. 68. Mix the ingredients in a 100 ml sterilized, dark glass bottle.

DOSAGE *Take 10 ml in 100 ml water twice a day before meals.*

CAUTION
• *This remedy should only be used for mild, stable conditions. Asthma can be life-threatening: seek professional help in severe cases. Do not suddenly stop using steroidal or other inhalants; their use should only be phased out gradually with professional help.*

Supplementary treatment
■ Use 5 drops of chamomile oil in a basin of boiling water as a steam inhalation (see p. 78) at the first hint of an attack.

Candidiasis

Candidiasis is the accelerated growth of yeast-like fungi, usually *Candida albicans*, which are naturally present in the gut. Candidiasis has been identified by some specialists as causing a wide variety of health problems, ranging from thrush and persistent urinary infections to panic attacks and chronic digestive disorders. Although some doctors remain sceptical, a low-sugar, yeast-free regime can help in many cases.

MARIGOLD & AGRIMONY TEA

Pot marigold is a good antifungal, both internally and externally, while agrimony helps to soothe the gut irritation caused by allergens and heal the mucous membranes.

~ INGREDIENTS ~

10 g dried echinacea root (*Echinacea angustifolia*)
600 ml water
10 g dried pot marigold petals (*Calendula officinalis*)
15 g dried agrimony leaves (*Agrimonia eupatoria*)

~ HOW TO MAKE THE TEA ~

1 Simmer the echinacea root in the water for 10 minutes to make a decoction.

2 Mix the pot marigold and agrimony in a teapot and pour on the freshly made decoction. Infuse for 10 minutes. Strain into a jug and cover. The surplus may be kept in a cool place or refrigerator for up to 48 hours.

DOSAGE *Drink a wineglass dose 3 times a day before meals until the infection clears. Do not sweeten the tea with honey or sugar while on a yeast-free diet – try a squeeze of fresh lemon juice or 1–2 drops of peppermint essence instead.*

Supplementary treatments

■ Garlic is an antifungal herb – take 1–2 x 200 mg capsules 3 times a day or use plenty of garlic in cooking.
■ Take 1 g evening primrose oil capsules and 1–2 capsules containing lactobacillus bacteria (e.g. *L. acidophilus* and *L. bifidus*) daily.
■ Avoid yeast-extracts, fungi-based foods (e.g. mycoproteins, mushrooms), sugars, dairy products, alcohol, refined carbohydrates, junk food and preserved foods. Avoid excessive amounts of fruit.
■ Candidiasis can give rise to a wide range of symptoms. Select infusions and additional treatments to match the pattern of symptoms. See pp. 116–17 for joint pain treatments and pp. 102–7 for digestive remedies.

Food intolerance

Food sensitivity often starts in childhood with the introduction of cow's milk, which is a protein alien to the developing digestive system. If possible, breastfeed babies for the first 4 months, or use non-cow's milk formulations. Food intolerance can cause chronic digestive disturbances, arthritis-like symptoms, eczema, asthma and ear problems. Eliminating the problem food is essential, in the meantime herbs can help repair the system and increase tolerance.

MARSHMALLOW & LEMON BALM TEA

Soothing marshmallow coats and protects the gut, and lemon balm is a carminative, ideal for digestive upsets.

~ INGREDIENTS ~

5 g dried marshmallow root (*Althaea officinalis*)
5 g fenugreek seeds (*Trigonella foenum-graecum*)
10 g dried *Dang Shen* (*Codonopsis pilosula*)
750 ml water
10 g dried or 30 g fresh lemon balm leaves
(*Melissa officinalis*)
10 g dried agrimony (*Agrimonia eupatoria*)

~ HOW TO MAKE THE TEA ~

1 Simmer the marshmallow, fenugreek and *Dang Shen* in the water for 15–20 minutes to make a decoction.

2 Put the lemon balm and agrimony in a teapot and pour on the freshly made decoction. Infuse for 10 minutes. Strain into a jug and cover.

DOSAGE *Drink a wineglass dose 4 times a day.*

Supplementary treatments

■ It is essential to identify the problem food. Seek professional help or try eliminating possible allergens from the diet: milk and milk products, wheat, red meat, salicylates, tomatoes, potatoes and peppers.

OVER-THE-COUNTER REMEDIES
Allergies

■ Look out for patent hayfever remedies that contain eyebright, ephedra (*Ma Huang*) or goldenseal.
■ Various remedies for candidiasis are on offer, although so far there is little evidence to support their claims. They may contain biotin, caprylic acid and derivatives, echinacea, evening primrose oil, linseed oil and tea tree oil.

DIGESTIVE PROBLEMS

WE ARE NOT ONLY WHAT WE EAT, but also what we digest. Keeping the digestive system in good working order is a vital part of staying healthy as failure to extract the necessary nutrients from food, or to excrete surplus wastes, can lead to all sorts of health problems, such as vitamin or mineral deficiencies, arthritic or skin problems associated with toxins lingering in the system, or headaches.

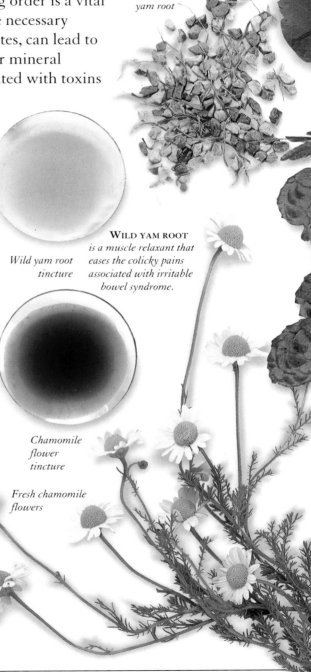

Fresh hop aerial parts

Dried wild yam root

Irritable bowel syndrome

Irritable bowel syndrome is a common label for a wide range of gastric symptoms, generally characterized by alternating diarrhoea and constipation, as well as flatulence, abdominal bloating and pain. It is commonly related to stress or food intolerance (see p. 101).

Wild yam root tincture

WILD YAM ROOT *is a muscle relaxant that eases the colicky pains associated with irritable bowel syndrome.*

—— *WILD YAM & CHAMOMILE MIXTURE* ——

Wild yam is an effective antispasmodic that helps to relax the gut and relieve the over-activity contributing to the problem. Hops and chamomile act as relaxants, while the bitterness of hops helps restore normal digestion.

~ INGREDIENTS ~
30 ml wild yam root tincture (*Dioscorea villosa*)
30 ml chamomile flower tincture (*Matricaria recutita*)
20 ml bistort tincture (*Polygonum bistorta*)
15 ml hop tincture (*Humulus lupulus*)
5 ml liquorice fluid extract (*Glycyrrhiza glabra*)

~ HOW TO MAKE THE MIXTURE ~
To make the individual tinctures, see p. 68. Pour the tinctures and fluid extract into a 100 ml sterilized, dark glass bottle and shake.

DOSAGE *Take 5 ml in 100 ml of warm water 3 times a day until symptoms ease.*

Chamomile flower tincture

Fresh chamomile flowers

CHAMOMILE FLOWERS *help to counter stress, which is often a factor in irritable bowel syndrome. They calm the nerves and the digestive system.*

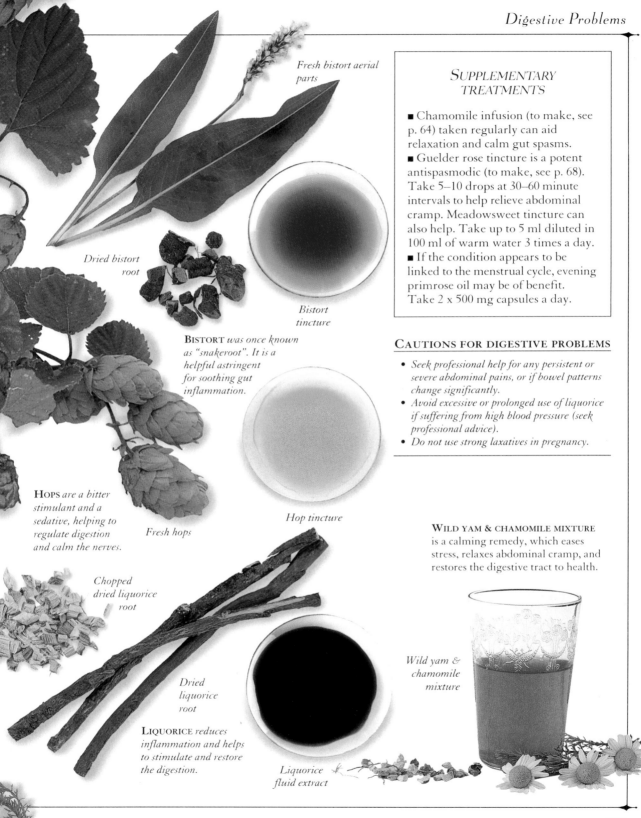

Fresh bistort aerial parts

Dried bistort root

Bistort tincture

BISTORT *was once known as "snakeroot". It is a helpful astringent for soothing gut inflammation.*

HOPS *are a bitter stimulant and a sedative, helping to regulate digestion and calm the nerves.*

Fresh hops

Hop tincture

Chopped dried liquorice root

Dried liquorice root

LIQUORICE *reduces inflammation and helps to stimulate and restore the digestion.*

Liquorice fluid extract

SUPPLEMENTARY TREATMENTS

■ Chamomile infusion (to make, see p. 64) taken regularly can aid relaxation and calm gut spasms.
■ Guelder rose tincture is a potent antispasmodic (to make, see p. 68). Take 5–10 drops at 30–60 minute intervals to help relieve abdominal cramp. Meadowsweet tincture can also help. Take up to 5 ml diluted in 100 ml of warm water 3 times a day.
■ If the condition appears to be linked to the menstrual cycle, evening primrose oil may be of benefit. Take 2 x 500 mg capsules a day.

CAUTIONS FOR DIGESTIVE PROBLEMS

- *Seek professional help for any persistent or severe abdominal pains, or if bowel patterns change significantly.*
- *Avoid excessive or prolonged use of liquorice if suffering from high blood pressure (seek professional advice).*
- *Do not use strong laxatives in pregnancy.*

WILD YAM & CHAMOMILE MIXTURE is a calming remedy, which eases stress, relaxes abdominal cramp, and restores the digestive tract to health.

Wild yam & chamomile mixture

Constipation

Failure to empty the bowels regularly can be linked to a lack of dietary fibre or to a sluggish digestion. In the West, it can take 72 hours for food to pass through us, as against an average of 12 in developing countries, where food is less highly processed.

— LIQUORICE & DANDELION DECOCTION —

Chronic constipation often suggests a sluggish digestion, which can be improved by bitter herbs that stimulate the liver and encourage production of digestive enzymes. Dandelion is a good liver tonic, while yellow dock has a gentle laxative action.

~ INGREDIENTS ~

10 g dried dandelion root (*Taraxacum officinale*)
5 g dried yellow dock root (*Rumex crispus*)
5 g dried liquorice root (*Glycyrrhiza glabra*)
5 g dried anise seeds (*Pimpinella anisum*)
750 ml water

~ HOW TO MAKE THE DECOCTION ~

1 Put the herbs in a pan and add the water.

2 Bring to the boil and simmer gently for 10 minutes, or until the volume has reduced by approximately one-third. Strain into a jug. Cover, and store in a cool place.

DOSAGE *Take a wineglass dose 3 times a day.*

CAUTIONS
- *Recurrent constipation can indicate more serious underlying health conditions. Seek professional advice before resorting to persistent or excessive use of laxatives.*
- *Do not use strong laxatives, e.g. senna or rhubarb, during pregnancy.*

Supplementary treatments
■ Take regular exercise and drink plenty of fluids, especially a glass of warm water first thing in the morning.
■ Isphagula husks and seeds can help to lubricate the bowel, easing the passage of dry, hard stools. Add a teaspoon of seeds to a cup of boiling water. Infuse for 10 minutes, stir well and drink the entire mix first thing in the morning.
■ Rhubarb root is a potent laxative. Take 10–20 drops of the tincture (to make, see p. 68) in 100 ml of warm water 3 times a day before meals for chronic problems. If pregnant, use butternut in the same way.
■ If tension is part of the problem, take 2–3 ml of guelder rose tincture in 100 ml of warm water before meals.

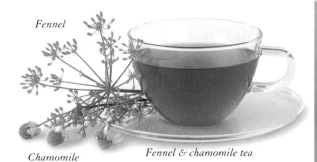

Fennel

Chamomile   *Fennel & chamomile tea*

Flatulence

Wind – travelling in either direction – can be a symptom of various digestive ailments, such as gastritis, gallbladder problems or irritable bowel syndrome (see p. 102). It can also be associated with poor diet, nervousness or stress. Carminative herbs after meals can help, but professional advice may be needed to identify the cause of the problem.

— FENNEL & CHAMOMILE TEA —

The calming and anti-inflammatory actions of fennel and chamomile provide a soothing mixture for the relief of wind. This is also a palatable after-dinner infusion, suitable for regular use.

~ INGREDIENTS ~

25 g dried fennel seeds (*Foeniculum officinalis*)
25 g dried chamomile flowers (*Matricaria recutita*)
10 g dried peppermint aerial parts (*Mentha piperita*)
water

~ HOW TO MAKE THE TEA ~

1 Mix the herbs and store in a dry, airtight container.

2 Put 2–3 teaspoonfuls of the mix in a tisane cup or small teapot. Add a cup of freshly boiled water and infuse for 5–10 minutes. Strain.

DOSAGE *Drink a cup regularly after meals.*

Supplementary treatments
■ Many culinary herbs aid digestion: add anise, dill, fennel or lemon balm to dishes, and cook with warm spices such as ginger, fenugreek, caraway or cayenne.
■ If symptoms are severe, massage the abdomen with a mixture of 2 drops of cinnamon or clove oil in 10 ml of sweet almond oil.

Diarrhoea

Diarrhoea, characterized by loose and frequent stools, is generally a symptom of imbalance rather than a primary disease. Food poisoning or bacterial infections are often responsible for sudden attacks, and the aim of treatment is to help the body to rid itself of toxins, rather than simply suppressing the symptoms.

TORMENTIL & MARSHMALLOW DECOCTION

This mixture of herbs and arrowroot is soothing and nutritious. Tormentil root is rich in tannins and highly astringent, helping to reduce inflammation, while marshmallow is soothing.

~ INGREDIENTS ~
1 tablespoon arrowroot
15 g dried tormentil root (*Potentilla erecta*)
10 g dried marshmallow root (*Althaea officinalis*)
5 g dried cinnamon bark (*Cinnamomum zeylanicum*)
750 ml water

~ HOW TO MAKE THE DECOCTION ~

1 Blend the arrowroot with a tablespoon of cold water to form a paste in a bowl or jug.

2 Simmer the herbs in the water for 10–15 minutes. Strain, return the liquid to the pan and bring to the boil.

3 Pour the boiling decoction over the blended arrowroot stirring well. Store the surplus in a cool place.

DOSAGE *Take a teacup dose 3 times a day until symptoms subside. Sweeten with honey if required.*

BISTORT & AGRIMONY TINCTURE

Diarrhoea can be a problem on holiday, with strange foods and unfamiliar bugs. This mixture is useful to pack in the luggage for emergencies. Both agrimony and bistort are astringent herbs, helpful for treating diarrhoea.

~ INGREDIENTS ~
25 ml bistort tincture (*Polygonum bistorta*)
35 ml agrimony tincture (*Agrimonia eupatoria*)
20 ml marshmallow tincture (*Althaea officinalis*)
10 ml *Lian Qiao* tincture (forsythia berries – *Forsythia suspensa*)
10 ml *Jin Yin Hua* (*Lonicera japonica*)

~ HOW TO MAKE THE TINCTURE ~

To make the individual tinctures, see p. 68. Mix the tinctures in a sterilized, dark glass bottle.

DOSAGE *Take 10 ml of the tincture in 100 ml of warm water 3 times a day when symptoms are acute. Repeat for up to 3 days.*

CAUTION
• *Seek professional help if diarrhoea persists for more than 2 or 3 days (or more than 24 hours in babies or toddlers); if it is accompanied by fever; or if there is blood or mucus in the stool.*

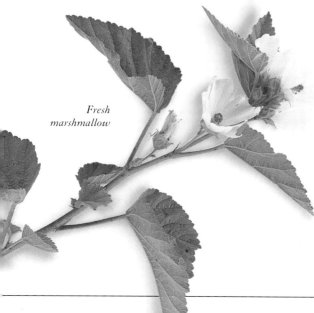

Fresh marshmallow

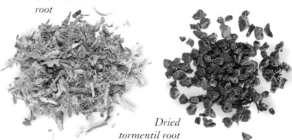

Dried marshmallow root

Dried tormentil root

Supplementary treatments
■ Drink cups of strong, cool, black Indian tea, without milk or sugar, to reduce inflammation in the gut.
■ Meadowsweet tincture (to make, see p. 68) can be very soothing for gut inflammation. Take 2 ml in warm water at hourly intervals up to 10 times a day.
■ An infusion (to make, see p. 64) of agrimo y can be helpful. Drink a cup 3 or 4 times a day.

Haemorrhoids

Haemorrhoids, or piles, are varicose veins in the wall of the rectum, frequently associated with constipation, liver imbalance or poor diet. They also may occur during pregnancy. They often bleed and may be inflamed. Increasing dietary intake of fruit and vegetables can help.

———— PILEWORT OINTMENT ————

In the Middle Ages the nodular roots of the lesser celandine plant reminded people of the appearance of piles – hence the traditional, alternative name for the herb. Pilewort is a very astringent plant, and can be extremely helpful for haemorrhoids.

~ INGREDIENTS ~

75 g dried pilewort leaves (*Ranunculus ficaria*)
500 ml sunflower oil
25 g beeswax
25 g anhydrous lanolin

~ HOW TO MAKE THE OINTMENT ~

1   Heat the pilewort and the oil in a double saucepan, or over a waterbath, for 3 hours to make an infused oil and strain the mixture through a jelly bag (see p. 73).

2   Meanwhile, melt the beeswax and anhydrous lanolin in a separate saucepan.

3   Add 100 ml of the warm infused oil to the melted wax mixture in the saucepan. Stir well and pour the ointment into sterilized jars before it starts to set.

APPLICATION *Gently rub the ointment on affected areas several times a day.*

Supplementary treatments

■ If the piles are irritant or bleeding, apply a little distilled witch hazel on cotton-wool to the affected area.
■ Drink an infusion (see p. 64) made from equal amounts of yarrow, linden flowers and melilot to help improve venous circulation.
■ Avoid constipation which exacerbates haemorrhoids – follow the recommendations on p. 104.

Gastritis

Gastritis or inflammation of the stomach lining is a common result of "over-indulgence" or upsetting foods, and can lead to nausea, vomiting, diarrhoea and heartburn. Symptoms are usually short-lived.

———— MEADOWSWEET TEA ————

Meadowsweet is a cooling and very soothing herb, which eases inflammation and helps to reduce acidic secretions in the stomach.

~ INGREDIENTS ~

25 g fresh meadowsweet (*Filipendula ulmaria*)
500 ml water

~ HOW TO MAKE THE TEA ~

Place the herb in a teapot. Add freshly boiled water and leave to infuse for 10 minutes. Strain the surplus into a covered jug and store in a cool place.

DOSAGE *Sip a large mugful of the mixture when symptoms are acute. Flavour with a little honey or liquorice juice if required. Repeat if necessary.*

CAUTION

• *Avoid excessive use of meadowsweet in cases of aspirin allergy.*

Supplementary treatments

■ Meadowsweet tincture (to make, see p. 68) can be taken as an alternative to the tea. Take 2 ml in warm water every hour while symptoms persist, up to 10 times a day.
■ Take 2–3 slippery elm capsules every couple of hours while symptoms are severe.
■ If the gastritis is linked to a hangover, take 5 ml of milk thistle tincture and 2 x 500 mg capsules of evening primrose oil. Repeat every 3 hours while symptoms continue for up to 12 hours.

Meadowsweet

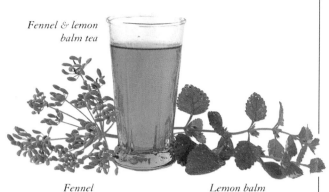

Fennel & lemon balm tea

Fennel   *Lemon balm*

Indigestion & heartburn

Eating too quickly, or while sitting awkwardly, can often lead to indigestion. If it is a regular problem, then some underlying digestive imbalance may be to blame. Heartburn is a common problem in pregnancy and obesity, and it can also be a side-effect of some orthodox medication.

FENNEL & LEMON BALM TEA

Both these herbs are very calming for the stomach, while lemon balm also helps relax the nerves if stress or anxiety is contributing to the problem.

~ INGREDIENTS ~
10 g dried fennel seeds (*Foeniculum officinalis*)
15 g dried, or 45 g fresh lemon balm leaves
(*Melissa officinalis*)
2–3 g dried cinnamon bark or a pinch of powdered
cinnamon (*Cinnamomum zeylanicum*)
500 ml water

~ HOW TO MAKE THE TEA ~
Place the herbs in a teapot. Add freshly boiled water and leave to infuse for 10 minutes. Strain the surplus into a covered jug and store in a cool place.

DOSAGE *Take a wineglass dose after meals as required.*

Supplementary treatments
■ Slippery elm capsules or 5 g of the powdered bark stirred into a cup of water can soothe heartburn.
■ Take carminative teas regularly. Try chamomile, peppermint, fennel or lemon balm (to make, see p. 64).

Nausea & vomiting

Nausea and vomiting are common symptoms of digestive upsets, fevers and migraines. Many people also suffer from nausea in early pregnancy, or when travelling.

GINGER CAPSULES

Ginger in almost any form is excellent for nausea and vomiting. Crystallized ginger, ginger beer, ginger wine, or even ginger biscuits, can all be useful if nothing else is available. The herb has been shown to be safe and effective, even in pregnancy.

~ INGREDIENTS ~
50 g powdered ginger (*Zingiber officinalis*)
size 00 gelatine or vegetarian capsules

~ HOW TO MAKE THE CAPSULES ~
1 Pour the powdered ginger into a saucer.

2 Separate the 2 halves of a capsule case and slide them together through the powder, scooping it into the capsule. Join the 2 halves together.

DOSAGE *Take 2 capsules every couple of hours while symptoms persist.*

Supplementary treatments
■ Tinctures of black horehound, chamomile, cloves, ginger or greater celandine can help nausea. Keeping remedies down can be a problem in cases of severe nausea and vomiting. Try placing a couple of drops of tincture on the tongue for rapid absorption.

OVER-THE-COUNTER REMEDIES
Digestive Problems

■ Senna leaves and pods are readily available in tablets and capsules for constipation. This herb should be taken on an occasional basis, as it works by irritating the digestive tract to encourage movement and excessive use can weaken the gut in the long-term. Avoid during pregnancy.
■ Slippery elm capsules are helpful for gastritis and indigestion. They are readily available from health food stores.
■ Many "after-dinner" herbal tea blends contain digestive stimulants that can help regulate activity. Herbs used commercially include: barberry, boldo leaves (a liver stimulant), dandelion and vervain.

CIRCULATORY DISORDERS

HIGH BLOOD PRESSURE and other circulatory problems are widespread in the developed world, due in part to sedentary lifestyles, diets that are over-rich in saturated animal fats, smoking and excessive stress. Regular exercise and a healthy diet can help, as can simple herbal remedies, such as garlic and oat bran to reduce blood cholesterol levels and linden to ease stress and combat atherosclerosis.

Poor circulation & chilblains

Poor circulation can be an inherited condition, although it is also common among the elderly and those who have become run down and exhausted. Cold weather may make things worse, because as small arteries constrict, blood flow is restricted, leading to blue fingers and toes, and chilblains.

—— GINGER & CINNAMON TEA ——

Herbs that stimulate the circulation, such as cinnamon and ginger, are generally hot and spicy. The Chinese regard Gui Zhi *(cinnamon twigs) as the most effective part of the herb for sending heat to the peripheries, but the more familiar cinnamon stick (made from the bark) can be substituted if twigs are unavailable.*

~ INGREDIENTS ~

15 g fresh ginger root, sliced (*Zingiber officinalis*)
10 g *Gui Zhi* (cinnamon twigs – *Cinnamomum cassia*)
10 g dried angelica root (*Angelica archangelica*)
700 ml water

~ HOW TO MAKE THE TEA ~

Heat the herbs and the water in a pan and simmer for 10–15 minutes. Strain into a covered jug. The surplus can be stored in a cool place for up to 48 hours.

DOSAGE *Drink a teacup dose while it is hot. Take a dose 3 times a day, reheating the tea each time.*

Supplementary treatments

■ Use arnica cream (to make, see p. 76) or drops of arnica tincture (to make, see p. 68) on unbroken chilblains.
■ Drink buckwheat infusion regularly (to make, see p. 64) or take rutin tablets to help strengthen the circulation.
■ Foot or hand baths can be helpful. Soak the affected part in hot water and a dessertspoon of mustard powder.

High blood pressure

Raised blood pressure needs professional investigation as it may be a sign of heart, liver or kidney disease. Many cases have no obvious cause and herbs can provide a valuable alternative to orthodox remedies.

— HAWTHORN & CHRYSANTHEMUM TEA —

Hawthorn helps to improve the coronary circulation, making the heart more efficient, while chrysanthemum flowers relax the heart and improve blood flow. This mixture is ideal for mild conditions.

~ INGREDIENTS ~

30 g dried hawthorn flowering tops
(*Crataegus oxyacantha*)
25 g *Ju Hua* (dried, prepared chrysanthemum flowers – *Chrysanthemum morifolium*)
25 g dried linden flowers (*Tilia europaea*)
20 g dried yarrow (*Achillea millefolium*)
water

~ HOW TO MAKE THE TEA ~

1 Mix the herbs and store in a dry, airtight container.

2 Place 2 teaspoons of the mix in a tisane cup or small teapot. Add a cup of freshly boiled water and infuse for 10 minutes. Strain.

DOSAGE *Drink a teacup dose 3 times a day.*

CAUTIONS

● *Omit the yarrow if pregnant. Maintain regular blood pressure checks and do not replace long-term orthodox medication with herbs without first consulting a doctor or herbal practitioner.*

Supplementary treatment

■ Eliminate tea, coffee and alcohol from the diet and avoid added salt. Take 400 IU vitamin E daily.

Varicose veins

Progress of the blood through the veins on its return to the heart depends largely on muscle contractions. Lack of exercise, pregnancy or obesity can make the return tortuous: vessel walls weaken and blood stagnates leading to varicose veins, which can be seen as twisted, swollen veins on the skin's surface.

—— *STINGING NETTLE & MELILOT TEA* ——

Herbs rich in silica, such as stinging nettle and horsetail, help to strengthen the vein walls, as do herbs such as shepherd's purse and buckwheat, which contain bioflavonoids.

~ INGREDIENTS ~

10 g dried stinging nettle (*Urtica dioica*)
10 g dried melilot (*Melilotus officinalis*)
10 g dried shepherd's purse (*Capsella bursa-pastoris*)
or buckwheat (*Fagopyrum esculentum*)
20 ml horsetail juice (*Equisetum arvense*)
500 ml water

~ HOW TO MAKE THE TEA ~

1 Use commercially prepared horsetail juice. Or make a decoction by simmering 60 g of fresh herb in 750 ml water for at least 3 hours, topping up the water as necessary.

2 Mix the dried herbs together in a teapot or lidded jug and add the freshly boiled water. Infuse for 15 minutes and strain.

3 Add the horsetail juice or 100 ml of the homemade decoction to the infusion and stir well.

DOSAGE *Take a wineglass dose 3 times a day before meals.*

Supplementary treatments

■ Raise the foot of the bed by 10–15 cm.
■ Use compresses (see p. 71) of chilled, distilled witch hazel or horsechestnut tincture (to make, see p. 68) to ease the discomfort of varicose veins.

Stinging nettle   *Melilot*

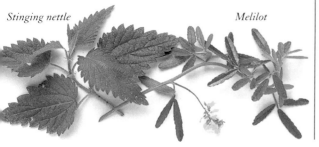

Iron-deficient anaemia

Iron is needed to make haemoglobin, which transports oxygen around the body in the blood. Its lack leads to anaemia characterized by fatigue, breathlessness, pallor, dizziness and rheumatic-like pains. Anaemia is common, especially among women with heavy periods.

—— *APRICOT IRON TONIC* ——

Apricots are rich in iron and are a good base for this tonic. Stinging nettles and dandelion are added to provide extra nutrients and to stimulate the liver.

~ INGREDIENTS ~

250 g fresh apricots
(wild or organically grown if possible)
500 ml water
1 litre red wine
250 g honey or sugar
100 ml stinging nettle tincture or juice (*Urtica dioica*)
50 ml dandelion root tincture (*Taraxacum officinale*)

~ HOW TO MAKE THE TONIC ~

1 To make the tinctures, see p. 68.

2 Put the apricots and water in a pan and bring to the boil. Transfer to a slow cooker and simmer for 12 hours.

3 Allow to cool and remove the stones. Blend in a food processor to produce a fruit pulp.

4 Add the red wine and herb tinctures and stir well. Store in sterilized, dark glass bottles for up to 3 months.

DOSAGE *Take 10 ml twice a day.*

CAUTION

• *Alcoholic mixtures should be avoided during pregnancy. Drink a cup of stinging nettle tea daily instead (to make, see p. 64).*

OVER-THE-COUNTER REMEDIES
Circulatory Disorders

■ For anaemia, try preparations rich in *Dang Gui* – often sold as a woman's tonic herb – to help nourish the blood. (*Dang Gui* should be avoided in pregnancy.)
■ *Ginkgo biloba* features as a circulatory herb in many over-the-counter mixtures. It is most useful as a remedy for cerebral circulation, but is also helpful for atherosclerosis which contributes to raised blood pressure.
■ Rutin tablets help to strengthen the circulation.

HEADACHES, MIGRAINES & NEURALGIA

HEADACHES ARE GENERALLY a sign that the body is out of balance. Those that seem to be focused behind the eyes are often characteristic of digestive problems. If they are in the front of the face, along the cheekbones, they may be part of a sinus disorder. Headaches that seem to start at the back of the neck and gradually creep over the skull are often tension-related. It is essential to treat the cause, which can mean changing eating habits or learning to relax.

GENERAL CAUTION
- *Seek professional advice if headaches are recurrent or sustained, as they can be a symptom of high blood pressure and other conditions.*

Tension headaches

Tension headaches start at the end of a long day or when stress begins to mount. If possible, take a break from the task in hand – go for a short walk, or spend a few minutes brewing a relaxing and soothing tea, and then take time to drink it slowly.

—— WOOD BETONY TEA ——
This relaxing mixture is based on wood betony, one of the most popular medicinal herbs in medieval times. The herb is a potent painkiller and relaxant.

~ INGREDIENTS ~
30 g dried wood betony (*Stachys betonica*)
10 g dried chamomile (*Matricaria recutita*)
10 g dried skullcap (*Scutellaria lateriflora*)
water

~ HOW TO MAKE THE TEA ~
1 Mix the herbs and store in a dry, airtight container.

2 Place 2 teaspoons of the mixed herbs in a tisane cup or small teapot. Add freshly boiled water and infuse for 5–10 minutes. Strain.

DOSAGE *Drink the tea while it is still warm. Take a teacup dose every hour until the headache subsides.*

Supplementary treatment
■ Take 2–3 drops of wood betony or lavender tincture (to make, see p. 68) on the tongue at the first sign of the headache. Repeat every 20–30 minutes while symptoms persist.

Sinus headaches

Thick catarrh blocking the sinus cavities in the skull around the nose, eyes and cheeks can lead to severe head pain, which is persistent in some cases. The pain can extend to the upper jaw, simulating toothache.

—— LAVENDER & PINE INHALATION ——
Steam inhalations are a good way to clear catarrh. This mixture contains potent essential oils, which reduce inflammation and infection.

~ INGREDIENTS ~
water
10 drops lavender oil (*Lavandula angustifolia*)
5 drops pine oil (*Pinus sylvestris*)
5 drops eucalyptus oil (*Eucalyptus globulus*)
5 drops thyme oil (*Thymus vulgaris*)

~ HOW TO USE THE INHALATION ~
1 Fill a large basin or mixing bowl with boiling water. Add the oils.

2 Lean over the water and cover the head and basin with a towel. Inhale the steam for 10 minutes. Repeat 2 or 3 times a day.
Note: Stay in a warm room for 30 minutes after each inhalation.

Supplementary treatments
■ If the sinus areas are not too painful, gently massage elderflower cream (to make, see p. 76) across the nose and cheeks 2 or 3 times a day. See also p. 90 for advice on treating sinusitis.

Migraines

Migraines are severe headaches that are often characterized by eye disturbances, such as flashing lights at the edges of the field of vision, as well as pins and needles in the arms and hands, and possibly nausea and vomiting. Stress, food intolerance and menstrual irregularities can all be trigger factors, and it is important to identify and treat the cause.

—— FEVERFEW & VALERIAN TINCTURE ——

Modern research has shown feverfew to be effective for treating migraine. Eating fresh leaves can prevent attacks, although the taste of the plant is extremely bitter.

~ INGREDIENTS ~

10 ml feverfew tincture (*Tanacetum parthenium*)
10 ml valerian tincture (*Valeriana officinalis*)
5 ml lavender tincture (*Lavandula angustifolia*)

~ HOW TO MAKE THE TINCTURE ~

To make the tinctures, see p. 68. Combine them in a sterilized dropper bottle.

DOSAGE *Drink 15–20 drops of the tincture in a little warm water. Repeat at 15–60 minute intervals while symptoms persist.*

CAUTIONS

• *Do not use feverfew if taking warfarin or other blood-thinning drugs.*
• *Feverfew can cause mouth ulcers. Do not use if this happens.*

Supplementary treatments

■ At the first signs of a migraine, massage a little of a mixture made from 20 drops lavender oil and 10 ml sweet almond oil into the nape of the neck and the temples.
■ See if a cold compress applied to the head eases the migraine (to make, see p. 71). If so, drinking lavender infusion can also help (to make, see p. 64). Other types of migraine respond to a hot towel on the forehead, in which case drink rosemary infusion (to make, see p. 64).

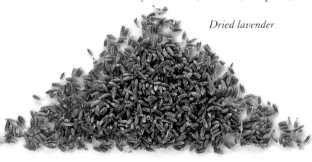

Dried lavender

Neuralgia

Inflammation of the facial nerves is often caused by chills and draughts, and occurs most commonly when the sufferer is tired and run down. The pain from the affected nerve, known as neuralgia, is severe and localized along the path of the nerve. The skin is usually extremely sensitive to touch.

—— ST JOHN'S WORT & LAVENDER TEA ——

St John's wort is a good restorative for the nervous system, helping to reduce inflammation, and lavender is a soothing herb that is frequently used to treat nervous complaints.

~ INGREDIENTS ~

15 g dried St John's wort (*Hypericum perforatum*)
10 g dried lavender flowers (*Lavandula angustifolia*)
500 ml water

~ HOW TO MAKE THE TEA ~

1 Mix the herbs together in a teapot.

2 Pour on the freshly boiled water and infuse for 10 minutes. Strain into a jug with a lid and store the surplus in a cool place for up to 48 hours.

DOSAGE *Slowly sip a large mug of the hot tea. Reheat the tea and continue sipping while the symptoms are severe.*

CAUTION

• *Seek professional help immediately if the area is very inflamed or hot, suggesting an acute infection, or if there is any paralysis or stiffness associated with the pain.*

Supplementary treatments

■ Very gently pat a little of a mixture made from 5 drops of lemon oil and 10 ml sweet almond oil on to the skin.
■ A hot compress soaked in an infusion made from St John's wort and vervain may help (to make, see p. 71).

OVER-THE-COUNTER REMEDIES
Headaches, Migraines & Neuralgia

■ For tension headaches, look out for combinations of relaxing herbs in capsules or tablets such as Californian poppy, chamomile, Jamaican dogwood, lemon balm, linden flowers, skullcap and valerian.
■ Feverfew tablets and capsules for migraines are readily available. Look for those that give a high parthenolide content or mention this key constituent on the pack.

MIND & EMOTIONS

STRESS IS A NORMAL part of life: the human body is designed to cope with regular rises in tension levels as the "flight or fight" hormone, adrenaline, prepares us for action. Problems arise when these peaks are sustained for too long. A perpetual state of alertness brings exhaustion and an inability to relax and wind down. It is important to tackle the underlying causes, as prolonged stress can cause emotional upsets and problems, such as depression and anxiety, and, if untreated, can start to affect bodily functions, leading, for example, to digestive disorders, headaches or lack of libido.

Coping with stress

Stress is blamed for a multitude of ills, but researchers believe that everyone needs a certain amount to function properly. Too much stress can be damaging, so it is important to learn when to take a break. Brewing a soothing herbal tea, and taking time to sip it slowly, is a good way to help the body unwind.

—— WOOD BETONY & LINDEN TEA ——

Wood betony was traditionally prescribed for the fearful and is a good restorative. Linden flowers, often used for heart-related disorders, are a nervine and can help prevent stress-related problems.

~ INGREDIENTS ~
20 g dried wood betony (*Stachys betonica*)
10 g dried linden flowers (*Tilia europaea*)
10 g dried chamomile flowers (*Matricaria recutita*)
10 g dried *gotu kola* (*Centella asiatica*)
water

~ HOW TO MAKE THE TEA ~

1 Mix the herbs and store in a dry, airtight container.

2 Put 2 teaspoons in a tisane cup or small teapot and add freshly boiled water. Infuse for 5–10 minutes. Strain.

DOSAGE *Drink a teacup dose 3 or 4 times a day as required.*

Supplementary treatments
■ Siberian ginseng improves the ability to cope with stress. Take 2–3 tablets a day several weeks before likely stressful periods, and continue until stress levels revert to normal.
■ Add 5 drops of lavender, basil or sandalwood oil to the bathwater at night (do not use basil oil in pregnancy).

Anxiety & tension

Irritability, tears, headaches and sleeplessness can all be signs of anxiety and tension. Identifying the cause of the problem is vital, as is learning to relax and unwind. Take 10 minutes a day to practise deep breathing exercises, use visualization tapes, or find time to meditate somewhere peaceful.

— SKULLCAP & PASSIONFLOWER MIXTURE —

Soothing herbal nervines encourage relaxation and reduce tensions. Skullcap is a restorative and relaxant, while passionflower has an effective sedative action.

~ INGREDIENTS ~
50 ml skullcap tincture (*Scutellaria lateriflora*)
25 ml passionflower tincture (*Passiflora incarnata*)
15 ml lemon balm tincture (*Melissa officinalis*)
10 ml pasque flower tincture (*Anemone vulgaris*)

~ HOW TO MAKE THE MIXTURE ~

To make the individual tinctures, see p. 68. Mix the tinctures together in a 100 ml sterilized, dark glass bottle.

DOSAGE *Take 5 ml in a little warm water when feeling anxious and tense. Repeat up to 5 times a day.*

Supplementary treatments
■ If symptoms include panic attacks, try massaging 5 drops of rose or neroli oil diluted in a teaspoon of sweet almond oil into the temples.
■ Bach Flower Remedies can be helpful for emotional tensions. Try red chestnut for worries about other people, elm for doubt in abilities and vervain for stress. Put 4 drops in a 10 ml dropper bottle of water and take 1–2 drops on the tongue at frequent intervals.

Depression

Everyone experiences emotional ups and downs, but when the downs turn into severe depression expert help is often needed to lift the spirits. Associated symptoms can include constipation, lack of concentration and a desire to withdraw from human company and say little.

—— LEMON BALM & OAT MIXTURE——

Oats are a good antidepressant and restorative for the nervous system and combine well with vervain. Lemon balm is a relaxant for the central nervous system. St John's wort is another effective nervous system remedy, widely used in Europe as an antidepressant.

~ INGREDIENTS ~
30 ml oat tincture (*Avena sativa*)
25 ml St John's wort tincture (*Hypericum perforatum*)
25 ml vervain tincture (*Verbena officinalis*)
15 ml lemon balm tincture (*Melissa officinalis*)
5 ml liquorice tincture (*Glycyrrhiza glabra*)

~ HOW TO MAKE THE MIXTURE ~
To make the individual tinctures, see p. 68. Mix the tinctures together in a 100 ml sterilized, dark glass bottle.

DOSAGE *Take 5–10 ml in a little warm water 3 times a day before meals.*

Supplementary treatments
■ Drink an infusion of wood betony and basil. Mix together equal amounts of dried basil and wood betony and store in a dry, airtight container. Make an infusion (see p. 64) using 1–2 teaspoons of the mix to a cup of water.
■ Use gorse, mustard or gentian Bach Flower Remedies. Put 4 drops of the flower remedy in a 10 ml dropper bottle of water and take 1–2 drops on the tongue at frequent intervals.
■ Add 5 drops of basil or sandalwood oil to the bathwater (do not use basil oil during pregnancy).

Insomnia

Over-excitement, worries, illness – the causes of sleeplessness are many. As always, identifying the contributing factors is vital. The pattern of insomnia is also important – is the problem an over-active mind preventing sleep, or restless, light sleep causing wakefulness in the early hours? In both cases relaxing in a warm bath before bed can often help.

—— NIGHTCAP & PASSIONFLOWER TEA ——

Californian poppies are sometimes known as "nightcap" and were once used as a sedative remedy by Native Americans. Like other poppies, they contain potent alkaloids, but these are far less powerful than the morphine of opium poppy, giving a gentle, soothing remedy that is safe to use, even for children.

~ INGREDIENTS ~
20 g dried Californian poppy (*Eschscholzia californica*)
15 g dried passionflower (*Passiflora incarnata*)
10 g dried wood betony (*Stachys betonica*)
5 g dried lavender flowers (*Lavandula angustifolia*)
water

~ HOW TO MAKE THE TEA ~
1 Mix the herbs and store in a dry, airtight container.

2 Put 2 teaspoons of the mix in a tisane cup and add freshly boiled water. Infuse for 5–10 minutes. Strain.

DOSAGE *Drink a cup about 30 minutes before going to bed. If required, make another cup and store in a vacuum flask to drink during the night.*

Supplementary treatments
■ Add 5 drops of lavender oil or 500 ml chamomile infusion (to make, see p. 64) to the bathwater at night.
■ If over-excitability is causing insomnia take 2 ml of cowslip flower tincture (to make, see p. 68) in a little warm water before going to bed.

OVER-THE-COUNTER REMEDIES
Mind & Emotions

■ Look out for relaxing remedies containing herbs such as chamomile, hops, Jamaican dogwood, pasque flower, passionflower, skullcap or vervain.
■ Valerian tablets, available from health food stores, can help to calm anxiety and help with sleeplessness.

■ Herbal infusions containing chamomile, linden or vervain are a valuable supplement to other theraputic approaches. Use instead of tea and coffee during the day.
■ Bach Flower Remedies are valuable for many different types of emotional problems.

MUSCLES, BONES & JOINTS

HERBAL REMEDIES can relieve the symptoms of creaking joints and aching bones and muscles, as well as treating the cause of the problem and encouraging healing. Long-term aches, such as arthritis, often respond to dietary treatment, while cleansing herbal remedies help alleviate the condition by clearing toxins from the system.

Backache & sciatica

Backache is one of the most common reasons for seeking medical help in the West. Finding the cause of the problem is important, as mechanical damage affecting discs or trapped nerves (as in sciatica) can often be helped by osteopathy or chiropractic treatments. Massage can help relieve aching muscles.

—— *LAVENDER & THYME RUB* ——

Lavender oil is a mild analgesic and can relieve many types of backache, while thyme is an antispasmodic that relaxes over-tense muscles. They can be combined with warming oils to soothe aches and pains.

~ INGREDIENTS ~
10 drops lavender oil
(*Lavandula angustifolia*)
10 drops thyme oil (*Thymus vulgaris*)
5 drops juniper oil (*Juniperus communis*)
10 drops eucalyptus oil (*Eucalyptus globulus*)
5 drops pine oil (*Pinus sylvestris*)
18 ml infused St John's wort oil
(*Hypericum perforatum*)

~ HOW TO MAKE THE RUB ~
Take care to use good quality oils (see p. 83). To make the infused St Johns's wort oil, see p. 73. Mix the oils in a 100 ml sterilized, dark glass bottle and shake well.

APPLICATION *Pour about a teaspoonful of the oil on to one palm and gently rub your hands together before massaging very gently into painful areas. Repeat at least twice a day.*

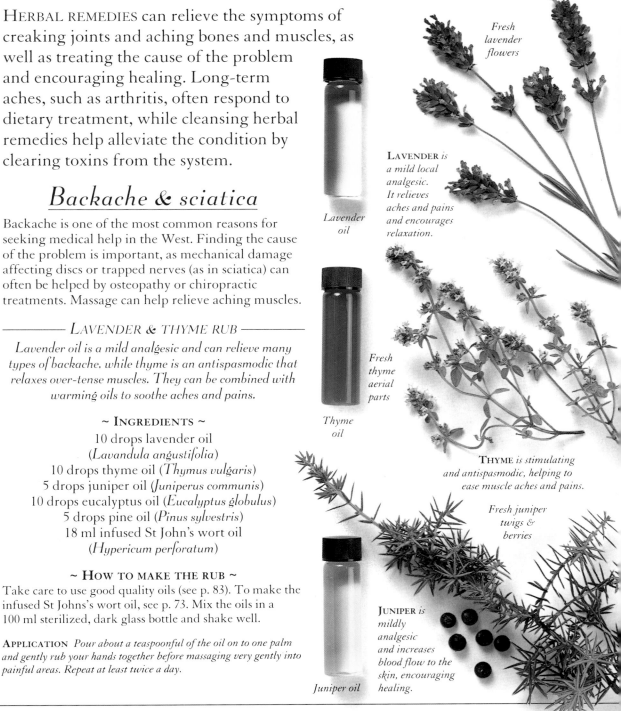

Fresh lavender flowers

Lavender oil

LAVENDER *is a mild local analgesic. It relieves aches and pains and encourages relaxation.*

Fresh thyme aerial parts

Thyme oil

THYME *is stimulating and antispasmodic, helping to ease muscle aches and pains.*

Fresh juniper twigs & berries

JUNIPER *is mildly analgesic and increases blood flow to the skin, encouraging healing.*

Juniper oil

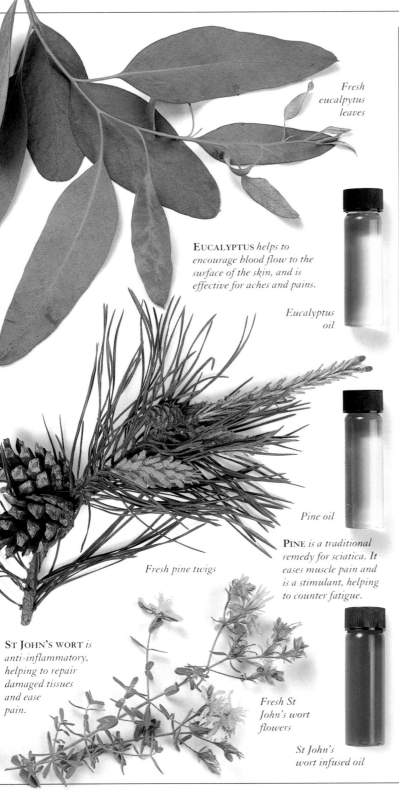

Fresh eucalyptus leaves

EUCALYPTUS *helps to encourage blood flow to the surface of the skin, and is effective for aches and pains.*

Eucalyptus oil

Pine oil

PINE *is a traditional remedy for sciatica. It eases muscle pain and is a stimulant, helping to counter fatigue.*

Fresh pine twigs

ST JOHN'S WORT *is anti-inflammatory, helping to repair damaged tissues and ease pain.*

Fresh St John's wort flowers

St John's wort infused oil

SUPPLEMENTARY TREATMENTS

■ A compress (see p. 71) soaked in 15 ml guelder rose tincture and 5 ml cinnamon tincture diluted in 100 ml hot water can help relieve backache. (To make the tinctures, see p. 68.)

■ Mix 2 ml each of St John's wort, guelder rose and willow bark tinctures and dilute with a little warm water. Sip 3 times a day.

■ For chronic conditions, drinking an infusion of St John's wort and valerian (to make, see p. 64) can help.

■ Consult a doctor if the pain starts with an accidental injury. Take homeopathic *Arnica* 6x tablets and repeat at hourly intervals for up to 12 hours to ease shock and trauma.

CAUTIONS FOR BACKACHE

- *Massage is not an appropriate treatment for inflammation or where there is any kind of injury. If in doubt always take professional advice.*
- *Painful areas of the body should be massaged gently.*
- *If sudden back pain does not clear within a few days, seek professional assistance.*

LAVENDER & THYME RUB relaxes tense muscles and relieves pain. It is ideal for soothing backache. Stored in a dark glass bottle, it will keep for about 3 months.

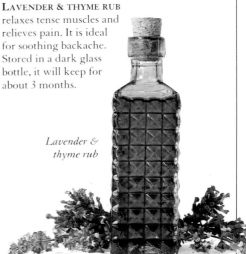

Lavender & thyme rub

Rheumatism

Also known as lumbago or fibrositis, muscular rheumatism (myalgia) is common from late middle age onwards. In this condition, the connective tissues and tendons associated with leg or arm muscles become inflamed. Warming rubs can often help to relieve the discomfort, and internal remedies are also useful when the condition is persistent.

—— BOGBEAN & MEADOWSWEET TEA ——

Bogbean is a wild, water plant, often found in bogs and shallow ponds. Meadowsweet also likes to grow in damp ditches and hedgerows. Both are anti-inflammatory and digestive stimulants. By stimulating and strengthening the digestion, the herbs help to clear the build-up of toxins that are frequently associated with muscle and joint disorders. They have a bitter taste, disguised in this remedy with liquorice extract.

~ INGREDIENTS ~

15 g dried bogbean leaves (*Menyanthes trifoliata*)
10 g dried meadowsweet (*Filipendula ulmaria*)
5 g dried yarrow (*Achillea millefolium*)
500 ml water
5 ml liquorice fluid extract (*Glycyrrhiza glabra*)

~ HOW TO MAKE THE TEA ~

1 Mix the dried herbs together in a teapot or jug and pour on 500 ml of freshly boiled water. Infuse for 10 minutes and strain.

2 Add the liquorice extract to the strained infusion and stir well. Store in a covered jug in a cool place.

DOSAGE *Take a wineglass dose 3 times a day, reheating each time.*

Supplementary treatments

■ Use a rub made from 10 drops each of lavender, marjoram, thyme and juniper oils in 20 ml of sweet almond oil on aching areas several times a day.
■ If pain prevents sleep, take 5 ml each of wild lettuce tincture and passionflower tincture in some warm water before going to bed (to make the tinctures, see p. 68).
■ Warm compresses can sometimes help: mix 10 ml arnica tincture, 20 ml guelder rose tincture and 20 ml angelica root tincture in 150 ml of hot water (to make the tinctures, see p. 68). Soak a pad in the the solution and apply to the painful area. Reheat the mixture for a fresh compress. *Caution: Do not use arnica on broken skin.*

Cramp

Muscle cramp can often be related to poor circulation and varicose veins, as well as stress, fatigue and mineral imbalance. It is also common during pregnancy. Sudden cramp in hot weather can be a sign of salt deficiency.

—— GUELDER ROSE & LAVENDER RUB ——

Another name for guelder rose is cramp bark – accurately describing its relaxing action. This rub is suitable for all kinds of muscle cramp.

~ INGREDIENTS ~

25 ml guelder rose tincture (*Viburnum opulus*)
2 ml lavender oil (*Lavandula angustifolia*)
2 ml marjoram oil (*Origanum vulgare*)
20 ml sweet almond oil

~ HOW TO MAKE THE RUB ~

To make the tincture, see p. 68. Mix the ingredients in a 50 ml sterilized, dark glass bottle and shake thoroughly.

APPLICATION *Apply a little of the rub to the affected area, and massage vigorously. Repeat, as required, shaking the bottle thoroughly each time.*

Frozen shoulder & tennis elbow

Frozen shoulder is a chronic stiffness of the shoulder joint, and tennis elbow is inflammation of the tendons on the outside of the elbow joint.

—— YARROW & ST JOHN'S WORT RUB ——

Yarrow and St John's wort are anti-inflammatory. They are used to help ease muscle tension.

~ INGREDIENTS ~

2.5 ml yarrow oil (*Achillea millefolium*)
2.5 ml lavender oil (*Lavandula angustifolia*)
20 ml infused St John's wort oil (*Hypericum perforatum*)

~ HOW TO MAKE THE RUB ~

To make the infused oil, see p. 73. Mix the oils in a 25 ml sterilized, dark glass bottle and shake well.

APPLICATION *Put a little on your fingers and massage well into aching elbows or stiff shoulders. Repeat 3 or 4 times a day.*

Gout

The painful, swollen joints of gout are caused by a build-up of uric acid crystals in the tissues. Rich food, too much alcohol and excessive amounts of shellfish or fatty fish can all exacerbate the problem, and should be avoided. Cutting out caffeine and giving up smoking can also help.

—— CELERY & HEATHER TEA ——

Successful treatment of gout requires diuretics, which help the condition by clearing excess uric acid from the system. Celery seed, heather flowers and yarrow all have effective diuretic actions.

~ INGREDIENTS ~
50 g dried celery seed (*Apium graveolens*)
15 g dried heather flowers (*Calluna vulgaris*)
15 g dried yarrow (*Achillea millefolium*)
250 ml water

~ HOW TO MAKE THE TEA ~

1 Mix the herbs and store in a dry, airtight container.

2 Put 2 teaspoons of the mix in a jug or teapot and add freshly boiled water. Infuse for 10 minutes and strain.

DOSAGE *Drink half while still warm. Reheat and take the other half later in the day. Make a fresh tea each day.*

Supplementary treatments
■ If the sufferer can bear it – a poultice of mashed cabbage leaf placed gently on the affected area can help. To make the poultice, see p. 71.
■ Eat plenty of asparagus, which is a good diuretic.
■ Devil's claw can help ease inflamed joints. Take 2 x 200 mg capsules of the herb 3 to 4 times a day (or follow the dosage instructions on the pack).

Osteoarthritis

Arthritis involves pain and swelling in the joints. It can be caused by general wear-and-tear (osteoarthritis) when usually just one or two joints are affected, or it can be an inflammatory disorder, affecting many joints (rheumatoid arthritis). The latter usually requires complex and extensive professional treatment, but osteoarthritis may respond to home remedies.

—— ST JOHN'S WORT & CELERY MIX ——

This combination of tinctures will help to cleanse the system, stimulate the circulation and digestion, and reduce inflammation.

~ INGREDIENTS ~
20 ml St John's wort tincture (*Hypericum perforatum*)
20 ml celery seed tincture (*Apium graveolens*)
15 ml bogbean tincture (*Menyanthes trifoliata*)
15 ml angelica root tincture (*Angelica archangelica*)
15 ml yellow dock tincture (*Rumex crispus*)
10 ml *Gui Zhi* tincture (cinnamon twigs – *Cinnamomum cassia*)
5 ml liquorice tincture (*Glycyrrhiza glabra*)

~ HOW TO MAKE THE MIX ~

To make the individual tinctures, see p. 68. Combine the tinctures in a sterilized, dark glass bottle and shake well.

DOSAGE *Take 5 ml in a little warm water 3 times a day.*

Supplementary treatments
■ Make a standard infusion (see p. 64) of equal parts of boneset and yarrow and take 3 times a day to encourage sweating, thereby helping to clear toxins.
■ Rub the affected part with 5 ml rosemary oil and 5 ml juniper oil in 50 ml infused comfrey oil (to make, see p. 72).

OVER-THE-COUNTER REMEDIES *Muscles, Bones & Joints*

■ Ready-made rubs for muscle, bone and joint ailments are widely available. Look for mixtures with birch, cajeput, camphor oil and extracts, eucalyptus, juniper, lavender, peppermint, pine, rosemary, thyme or wintergreen.
■ Devil's claw is a potent anti-inflammatory remedy that has become widely available in the past few years. It is either very effective or seems to have no impact at all. Take for at least 6 weeks (following the instructions on the pack) before abandoning the treatment.
■ When buying over-the-counter remedies, look for those that contain combinations of angelica, black cohosh, bogbean, burdock, celery seed, lignum vitae resin, meadowsweet, pokeroot, stinging nettles, white willow, yarrow and yellow dock. These are herbs that cleanse the system, soothe inflammation and gently stimulate the digestion.

MALE PROBLEMS

IN TRADITIONAL CHINESE medicine, male sexual energy is closely associated with the kidneys, and tonics for this organ are often given to increase fertility and vigour. Problems with the prostate gland are one of the most widespread male disorders: in the West, orthodox treatment usually involves surgery or hormone therapy. Although herbs are no substitute for long-term medication, they provide gentle remedies suitable for mild conditions of both short-term infections and of chronic disorders.

Prostate disorders

The prostate gland sits beneath the bladder. It can become infected and inflamed (a condition known as prostatitis), and is commonly enlarged in older men, leading to difficulties with urination.

– *SAW PALMETTO & SIBERIAN GINSENG MIX* –

Saw palmetto has long been used as a sexual tonic. Modern research has confirmed its effectiveness at treating prostate problems – both for inflammation and enlargement. The mix can be used in both cases.

~ INGREDIENTS ~

40 ml saw palmetto tincture (*Serenoa repens*)
35 ml Siberian ginseng tincture
(*Eleutherococcus senticosus*)
25 ml echinacea tincture (*Echinacea angustifolia*)

~ HOW TO MAKE THE MIX ~

To make the individual tinctures, see p. 68. Mix the tinctures together in a 100 ml sterilized, dark glass bottle and shake well.

DOSAGE *Take 5 ml in half a tumbler of warm water 3 times a day. Increase to 10 ml in acute stages of prostatitis.*

CAUTIONS
• *Medical examination is recommended for prostate disorders because of the risk of prostate cancer.*
• *Do not stop taking long-term medication for prostate problems without first taking professional advice.*

Supplementary treatments
■ Make an infusion (see p. 64) using 10 g each of dried white deadnettle, cornsilk and pellitory-of-the-wall as a healing diuretic tea to help counter prostate enlargement.
■ Take 500 mg of evening primrose oil daily.

Urethritis

When infections invade the urinary tract the urethra can become inflamed, causing discharge and pain on passing urine. It is important to seek professional medical help, particularly if symptoms are severe. Urethritis can be associated with sexually-transmitted diseases, in which case the sufferer will be referred to a specialist clinic. The following remedy and self-help measures can alleviate the symptoms.

——— *BUCHU & COUCHGRASS TEA* ———

The South African buchu bush has diuretic and antiseptic properties and is gently stimulating for the kidneys, while common couchgrass rhizomes provide mucilages to soothe and heal the affected area.

~ INGREDIENTS ~
50 g dried buchu leaves (*Barosma betulina*)
30 g dried couchgrass rhizome (*Agropyron repens*)
20 g dried cornsilk (*Zea mays*)
water

~ HOW TO MAKE THE TEA ~

1 Mix the herbs and store in a dark, airtight container.

2 Put 2 teaspoons of the mix in a tisane cup or small teapot and pour on a cup of freshly boiled water. Infuse for 10 minutes and strain.

DOSAGE *Drink a teacup dose up to 6 times a day during the acute stage of infection.*

Supplementary treatments
■ Drink plenty of fluids, adding a pinch of baking soda to each glass of water to help reduce the acid content of the urine. Barleywater can be a particularly soothing drink.
■ Take 2 x 200 mg echinacea capsules 3 times a day.

Infertility

Male infertility is often associated with a low sperm count. Recent Danish research – albeit with only a small sample of men – suggests that modern "junk" foods and high levels of pesticides in food can be contributory factors. Eating organically grown produce, cutting out alcohol, caffeine and smoking, and wearing loose clothing can all help.

—— *HE SHOU WU & CINNAMON WINE* ——

He Shou Wu, or "fleeceflower", has been used as a reproductive energy tonic by the Chinese for generations. Taoist sages reputedly lived for centuries by taking the herb and it is traditionally used to increase sperm count.

~ INGREDIENTS ~
250 g dried *He Shou Wu* (*Polygonum multiflorum*)
150 g dried cinnamon bark (*Cinnamomum zeylanicum*)
100 g dried liquorice root (*Glycyrrhiza glabra*)
1–2 litres red wine

~ HOW TO MAKE THE WINE ~

1 Put all the herbs into a large vinegar vat, rum pot or similar crockery pot.

2 Pour on the red wine to fill the pot and cover the herbs completely.

3 Leave the mixture to steep for 10–14 days.

DOSAGE *Take a sherry glass dose of the mixture daily, topping up the red wine to keep the herbs covered.*

Note: The mixture will last for several months if it is kept well covered with wine. Discard if there is any sign of mould on the herbs.

Supplementary treatments
■ Take 2–3 garlic pearls and 500 mg ginseng capsules daily.
■ Ensure adequate intake of vitamins B-complex and E and top up zinc levels by eating pumpkin seeds regularly.
■ If stress may be contributing to the problem, take skull-cap, vervain, linden or chamomile infusions (see p. 64).

Impotence

Stress, exhaustion and excessive alcohol can all contribute to sexual problems, with low libido and difficulties with intercourse. Herbs have been used as aphrodisiacs in all cultures for centuries, and both Chinese and Ayurvedic medicine make a contribution with herbs such as *Wu Wei Zi* (schizandra berries) and *ashwagandha* (withania roots), which may be found in patent remedies.

—— *DAMIANA & CINNAMON TEA* ——

Damiana was traditionally used in South America as a potent aphrodisiac – indeed, its botanical name was once Turnera aphrodisiaca. *Schizandra has been used for centuries in China as a sexual tonic suitable for both men and women, enhancing staying power and vigour.*

~ INGREDIENTS ~
10 g dried cinnamon bark (*Cinnamomum zeylanicum*)
10 g *Wu Wei Zi* (dried schizandra berries – *Schisandra chinensis*)
15 g dried damiana leaf (*Turnera diffusa*)
500 ml water

~ HOW TO MAKE THE TEA ~

1 Mix the cinnamon, *Wu Wei Zi* and water in a pan and simmer for 15 minutes to make a decoction.

2 Put the damiana leaf in a teapot and pour on the simmering decoction.

3 Infuse for a further 10 minutes and strain. Store in a covered jug in a cool place.

DOSAGE *Drink a wineglass dose 3 times a day before meals.*

Supplementary treatments
■ Try body massage with essential oils before intercourse – jasmine, ylang ylang, rose, patchouli and sandalwood all have an aphrodisiac effect. Use 5 drops of essential oil of any of these in 5 ml of sweet almond oil.

OVER-THE-COUNTER REMEDIES Male Problems

■ Herbal aphrodisiacs come in all shapes and sizes – not all efficacious or containing even remotely suitable herbs. Look for remedies that include: *Bu Gu Zhi* (psoralea berries), damiana, *Dang Gui* (Chinese angelica), ginseng, *He Shou Wu* (fleeceflower root) and saw palmetto.

■ Herbal diuretics and urinary antiseptics are widely available in blends or teabags. Look for those containing bearberry, buchu, celery seed, cleavers, cornsilk, couch-grass, dandelion and yarrow. Avoid long-term use of diuretics containing juniper, which can irritate the kidneys.

FEMALE PROBLEMS

OLD HERBALS ARE FULL OF remedies for gynaecological problems –
many of them concerned with improving fertility, regulating periods
or easing childbirth (a life-threatening situation in days gone by).
Today, Western medicine tends to blame hormonal deficiencies
for many disorders, while the Chinese focus on energy imbalance
in organs associated with the female reproductive system,
and treat menstrual problems with liver tonics and
menopausal disorders with kidney remedies.

Heavy periods

Excessive bleeding is a common menstrual problem. It is
important to consult a doctor or professional herbalist to ensure
that no significant causes – such as fibroids or
endometriosis – are involved. Heavy bleeding often
leads to anaemia, so eat plenty of iron-rich foods.

LADY'S MANTLE & SHEPHERD'S PURSE TEA

*Lady's mantle, like other members of the rose
family, is a good astringent. It also helps regulate
menstrual imbalances. Shepherd's purse – also known as
"mother's hearts" – is useful for reducing excess bleeding.*

~ INGREDIENTS ~
20 g dried lady's mantle (*Alchemilla vulgaris*)
10 g dried shepherd's purse (*Capsella bursa-pastoris*)
10 g dried raspberry leaves (*Rubus idaeus*)
5 g dried pot marigold petals (*Calendula officinalis*)
5 g dried mugwort leaves (*Artemisia vulgaris*)
500ml water

~ HOW TO MAKE THE TEA ~
1 Mix the dried herbs together. Reserve one half
for the following day, storing it in a dry, airtight
container. Place the other half in a teapot or jug.

2 Add the freshly boiled water.

3 Infuse for 10 minutes and strain. Store the surplus
in a covered jug in a cool place.

DOSAGE *The tea may be taken daily for a few months as a preventative
measure. Drink a teacup dose 3 times a day, reheating if preferred.*

*Fresh lady's
mantle aerial
parts*

LADY'S MANTLE *as its name suggests, is a
traditional women's remedy. It
is widely used
in Europe.*

*Dried lady's
mantle aerial
parts*

*Fresh
shepherd's
purse aerial
parts*

*Dried shepherd's
purse aerial parts*

SHEPHERD'S PURSE *is highly
valued in both Eastern and
Western herbal repertoires for
its astringent properties.*

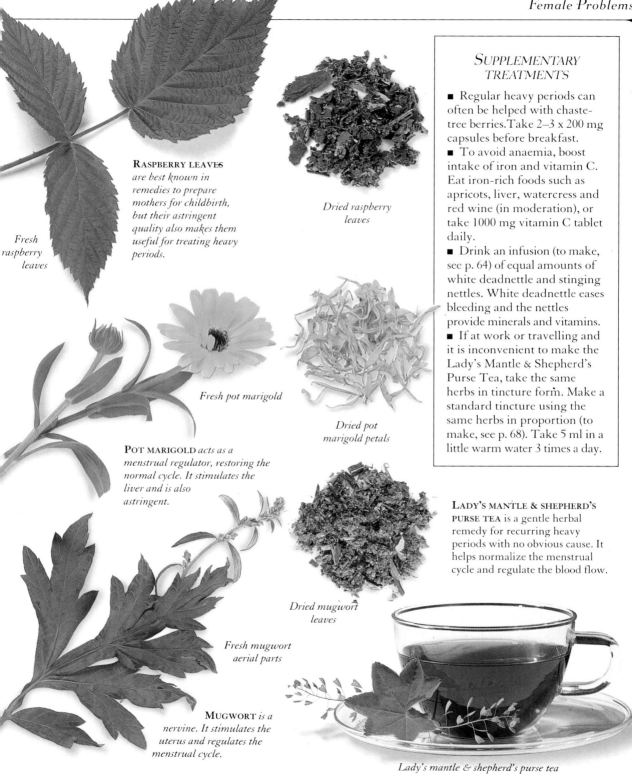

RASPBERRY LEAVES
are best known in remedies to prepare mothers for childbirth, but their astringent quality also makes them useful for treating heavy periods.

Dried raspberry leaves

Fresh raspberry leaves

SUPPLEMENTARY TREATMENTS

■ Regular heavy periods can often be helped with chaste-tree berries. Take 2–3 x 200 mg capsules before breakfast.

■ To avoid anaemia, boost intake of iron and vitamin C. Eat iron-rich foods such as apricots, liver, watercress and red wine (in moderation), or take 1000 mg vitamin C tablet daily.

■ Drink an infusion (to make, see p. 64) of equal amounts of white deadnettle and stinging nettles. White deadnettle eases bleeding and the nettles provide minerals and vitamins.

■ If at work or travelling and it is inconvenient to make the Lady's Mantle & Shepherd's Purse Tea, take the same herbs in tincture form. Make a standard tincture using the same herbs in proportion (to make, see p. 68). Take 5 ml in a little warm water 3 times a day.

Fresh pot marigold

Dried pot marigold petals

POT MARIGOLD *acts as a menstrual regulator, restoring the normal cycle. It stimulates the liver and is also astringent.*

Dried mugwort leaves

LADY'S MANTLE & SHEPHERD'S PURSE TEA is a gentle herbal remedy for recurring heavy periods with no obvious cause. It helps normalize the menstrual cycle and regulate the blood flow.

Fresh mugwort aerial parts

MUGWORT *is a nervine. It stimulates the uterus and regulates the menstrual cycle.*

Lady's mantle & shepherd's purse tea

Pre-menstrual syndrome

Western medicine usually describes pre-menstrual syndrome (PMS) in terms of hormone imbalance, while Oriental theories define it in terms of energy imbalance or stagnation. Typical symptoms include emotional upsets, irritability, breast tenderness, food cravings and digestive irregularities. Symptoms ease when menstruation starts. Relaxation and avoiding stimulants, such as caffeine, can help.

—— DANG GUI & PAEONY DECOCTION ——

This is based on a classical Chinese formula called "free and easy", which is often given to relieve the energy blocks contributing to PMS. Most of the herbs act on the liver, an organ associated with the female reproductive system.

~ INGREDIENTS ~

20 g *Dang Gui* (Chinese angelica – *Angelica sinensis*)
20 g *Bai Shao* (white paeony root – *Paeonia lactiflora*)
5 g *Chen Pi* (dried tangerine peel – *Citrus reticulata*)
5 g dried liquorice root (*Glycyrrhiza glabra*)
2 g fresh ginger root (*Zingiber officinalis*)
10 g dried vervain (*Verbena officinalis*)
2 g dried peppermint (*Mentha piperita*)
1 litre water

~ HOW TO MAKE THE DECOCTION ~

1 Simmer the *Dang Gui*, *Bai Shao*, *Chen Pi*, liquorice and ginger roots and the water in a pan for 15–20 minutes.

2 Put the vervain and peppermint into a teapot. Strain the simmering decoction on to the herbs. Infuse for 10 minutes, strain into a jug, and store in a cool place.

DOSAGE *The tea may be taken daily for a few months as a preventative measure. Drink a wineglass dose up to 5 times a day.*

Supplementary treatments
■ Take 10–20 drops of chaste-tree berry tincture each morning before breakfast (to make the tincture, see p. 68).
■ To ensure adequate intake of essential fatty acids, take 1 g daily of evening primrose or borage oils.

Period pain

There are various types of period pain: cramp when menstruation starts; heavy, nagging pains of stagnation beforehand; and spasmodic aches before bleeding. In many cases exercise can bring relief, and a brisk walk can be more beneficial than curling up with a hotwater bottle. Relaxation, a healthy sex life and avoiding stimulants, such as caffeine, may also help.

—— BLACK HAW TINCTURE ——

One of the best remedies for period cramps is black haw bark – a relaxing herb that has a specific action on the uterus. It works very well when taken on its own, but here it is combined with St John's wort, a restorative nerve tonic and pasque flower, which has antispasmodic properties.

~ INGREDIENTS ~

15 ml black haw bark tincture (*Viburnum prunifolium*)
2.5 ml St John's wort tincture (*Hypericum perforatum*)
2.5 ml pasque flower tincture (*Anemone vulgaris*)

~ HOW TO MAKE THE TINCTURE ~

To make the individual tinctures, see p. 68. Combine the tinctures in a sterilized, dark glass bottle.

DOSAGE *Take the whole quantity in a tumbler of warm water when period cramps start. Repeat up to 3 times a day as required.*

Supplementary treatments
■ To encourage relaxation, drink an infusion made from equal parts of dried St John's wort, raspberry leaves and skullcap (to make the infusion, see p. 64).
■ Dilute 10 drops each of cypress, marjoram and rosemary oil in 20 ml of sweet almond oil and gently massage into the abdomen.

Ingredients for Dang Gui & paeony decoction

Fresh vervain

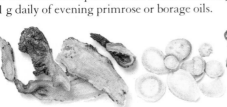

Dang Gui   Bai Shao   Chen Pi   *Fresh peppermint*   *Dried liquorice root*   *Fresh ginger root*

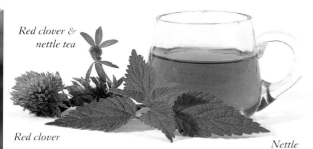

*Red clover &
nettle tea*

Red clover

Nettle

Menopause

As women age, hormone levels fall, until there are insufficient amounts to trigger the usual monthly menstruation, at which point ovulation and regular periods come to an end. Hormone levels continue to wax and wane, however, and menopausal women may experience symptoms similar to pre-menstrual syndrome. Menopausal problems can include hot flushes, night sweats, palpitations, vaginal dryness, sore eyes and emotional upsets.

—— HE SHOU WU & VERVAIN MIX ——

In Chinese tradition, menopausal problems are associated with run-down kidney energies, so tonics such as He Shou Wu that act on those organs are prescribed. Vervain is a good liver tonic and sedative to calm emotional upsets, while sage and wild yam help with more symptomatic menopausal problems.

~ INGREDIENTS ~

30 ml *He Shou Wu* tincture (fleeceflower root –
Polygonum multiflorum)
20 ml vervain tincture (*Verbena officinalis*)
20 ml sage tincture (*Salvia officinalis*)
15 ml wild yam root tincture (*Dioscorea villosa*)
10 ml lavender tincture (*Lavandula angustifolia*)
5 ml liquorice tincture (*Glycyrrhiza glabra*)

~ HOW TO MAKE THE MIX ~

To make the individual tinctures, see p. 68. Mix the tinctures and store in a 100 ml sterilized, dark glass bottle.

DOSAGE *Take 5 ml in a tumbler of warm water 3 times a day before meals.*

Supplementary treatments

■ If palpitations are a problem, make an infusion with 10 g each of dried motherwort, hawthorn tops and mugwort to 500 ml freshly boiled water (to make the infusion, see p. 64). Take a wineglass dose 3 times a day.
■ Apply vitamin E oil direct to the vagina to ease dryness. Regular sexual intercourse will help maintain a healthy vaginal lining.
■ For hot flushes and night sweats, make an infusion with 15 g each of dried sage and dried mugwort to 500 ml freshly boiled water (to make the infusion, see p. 64). Take a wineglass dose 3 times a day. Alternatively take a 200 mg goldenseal capsule 2 or 3 times a day (to make the capsules, see p. 70).

Infertility

The struggle to conceive can become a full-time preoccupation for many people. Modern fertilization techniques have done much to help. Herbs can improve general health and readiness for conception but, in general, they should be seen as supporting other approaches, rather than a remedy in themselves.

—— RED CLOVER & NETTLE TEA ——

Red clover is a good cleansing remedy, reputedly containing oestrogen-like compounds, while nettles are nourishing for the whole body. Peppermint is a good sexual stimulant and marigold strengthens the reproductive organs.

~ INGREDIENTS ~

45 g dried red clover flowers (*Trifolium pratense*)
25 g dried stinging nettle (*Urtica dioica*)
10 g dried peppermint (*Mentha piperita*)
20 g dried pot marigold petals (*Calendula officinalis*)
water

~ HOW TO MAKE THE TEA ~

1 Mix the herbs and store in an airtight, dark jar.

2 Place 2 teaspoons in a tisane cup or small teapot and add a cup of freshly boiled water. Infuse for 10 minutes and strain.

DOSAGE *Drink a teacup dose 2 or 3 times a day.*

Supplementary treatments

■ Take 5 drops of false unicorn tincture daily in a little warm water (to make the tincture, see p. 68).
■ Look for patent remedies based on *Dang Gui,* a herb that stimulates the reproductive system.
■ Chronic low-grade infections such as recurring thrush or cystitis can affect fertility. Take the remedies suggested for these conditions (see pp. 124 & 127) and boost the immune system by taking a 200 mg echinacea capsule 3 times a day.

Loss of libido

As with men, loss of sexual desire can be caused by a number of factors including exhaustion, stress and and an excess of stimulants such as caffeine. The rhythm of the menstrual cycle also plays a part, with libido often rising in mid-cycle, falling, and rising again just before bleeding starts. Stimulating herbal tonics can often help to counter loss of libido; learning to relax is also very important.

—— RASPBERRY & ROSEMARY TEA ——

As well as herbs that have a specific reputation as aphrodisiacs, sexual energies can be generally improved with nourishing, stimulating herbs. Nettle is rich in minerals and vitamins, rosemary is stimulating and raspberry leaves help to relax the reproductive organs.

~ INGREDIENTS ~
40 g dried raspberry leaves (*Rubus idaeus*)
20 g dried stinging nettles (*Urtica dioica*)
15 g dried rosemary (*Rosmarinus officinalis*)
15 g dried chaste-tree berries (*Vitex agnus-castus*)
10 g dried peppermint (*Mentha piperita*)
water

~ HOW TO MAKE THE TEA ~

[1] Mix the herbs and store in an airtight, dark jar.

[2] Place 2 teaspoons of the mixture in a tisane cup or small teapot. Add a cup of freshly boiled water and infuse for 10 minutes. Strain.

DOSAGE *Drink a teacup dose 2 or 3 times a day.*

Supplementary treatments
■ Chaste-tree berries can raise women's hormone activity and enhance sexuality. In addition to the tea, take 10–20 drops of tincture (to make, see p. 68) in warm water before breakfast.
■ Use essential oils in massage before intercourse – try 5–10 drops of jasmine, sandalwood, rose, ylang ylang, clary or neroli in 10 ml of sweet almond oil.
■ Drink a sherry glass daily of tonic wine made with *Wu Wei Zi* (schizandra berries). To make, see p. 69.
■ Relaxing herbs can help if tension is a problem. Make a standard infusion (see p. 64) using equal parts of skullcap, vervain and wood betony.
■ Stimulating herbs can improve vitality. Take 5–10 drops of ginger or cinnamon tinctures in warm water daily.

Vaginal infections

Vaginal secretions and the friendly bacteria they harbour usually prevent infections taking hold, but the quality of vaginal secretions can change as a result of a number of factors such as taking contraceptive pills, stress, general infections, antibiotic treatments or food intolerance. These give rise to conditions in which vaginal infections can develop. Thrush, a fungal infection characterized by a white discharge and itching, is one of the most common problems.

—— MARIGOLD & TEA TREE PESSARIES ——

Pot marigold is a useful antifungal and tea tree is one of the most effective herbal antiseptics available.

~ INGREDIENTS ~
20 g cocoa butter
10 drops pot marigold oil (*Calendula officinalis*)
10 drops tea tree oil (*Melaleuca alternifolia*)
5 drops thyme oil (*Thymus vulgaris*)

~ HOW TO MAKE THE PESSARIES ~

[1] Melt the cocoa butter in a double saucepan or a bowl over hot water.

[2] Make and lubricate foil shapes or a pessary mould as described on p. 70.

[3] Remove the cocoa butter from the heat and add the oils. Stir well and pour into the pessary mould or foil shapes. Allow to set (which takes about 4 hours). Remove from the mould or foil shapes. Store in a cool place in an airtight jar or pot lined with greaseproof paper.

APPLICATION *Insert a pessary into the vagina at night and repeat in the morning while the infection persists.*

OVER-THE-COUNTER REMEDIES
Female Problems

■ Look for patent remedies containing *Bai Shao* (white paeony) or *Dang Gui* (Chinese angelica), which can ease many menstrual disorders.
■ Evening primrose oil or other oils that are rich in essential fatty acids (e.g. borage, walnut, linseed or blackcurrant) can help menstrual problems.
■ For menopausal problems, remedies based on blue cohosh, *Dang Gui*, false unicorn root, goldenseal, *He Shou Wu*, *Nu Zhen Zi*, or sage, may be helpful.
■ Chaste-tree berry tablets are useful for many disorders.

PREGNANCY & CHILDBIRTH

HERBAL REMEDIES HAVE been used by generations of women to ease problems associated with pregnancy and childbirth. Many provide a safe alternative to orthodox remedies, but should still be used with respect during pregnancy. See the general caution on p. 126. There are herbal remedies available for common ailments that are particularly suitable for pregnant women. These include American ginseng as an energy tonic, butternut for constipation and nettle tea for anaemia (see pp. 104 and 109).

Morning sickness

Nausea and vomiting are common in early pregnancy, beginning in the third or fourth week and lasting up to three months. Occasionally they persist throughout pregnancy, and sufferers may need hospital treatment. Sufferers should consult a doctor if sickness is severe.

—— SIMPLE TINCTURES ——

Placing a few drops of tincture on the tongue is often the best way to take remedies when feeling nauseous.

~ TINCTURES ~
10 ml ginger tincture (*Zingiber officinalis*)
10 ml chamomile tincture (*Matricaria recutita*)
10 ml *Chen Pi* tincture (*Citrus reticulata*)
10 ml black horehound tincture (*Ballota nigra*)
10 ml peppermint tincture (*Mentha piperita*)
10 ml lemon balm tincture (*Melissa officinalis*)

~ HOW TO TAKE THE TINCTURES ~
To make the tinctures, see p. 68. Put each one into a separate 10 ml sterilized, dark glass dropper bottle.

DOSAGE *Place 2–3 drops of the chosen tincture on the tongue at the first sign of nausea. There is no simple rule for treating morning sickness and sufferers should experiment to discover which tincture suits them best, and vary the remedies as required.*

Supplementary treatments
■ Morning sickness can be related to digestive problems. Take 1–2 x 200 mg slippery elm capsules daily.
■ To encourage relaxation, sip an infusion (to make, see p. 64) of 35 g dried lemon balm, 15 g dried skullcap, 10 g dried lavender and 10 g dried peppermint, in teacup doses.
■ Ginger is very effective for morning sickness. Take 1 g per day in capsule form, or chew crystallized ginger.

Fluid retention (oedema)

Swollen ankles and puffiness of the hands or face are common problems in pregnancy. The growing baby sometimes upsets the protein balance of the blood, causing expectant mothers to retain as much as 5–6 litres of fluid. Simple oedema can be relieved with rest, eating grapes, asparagus and apples, limiting salt intake and the use of gentle diuretic teas to encourage elimination of excess fluid.

—— CORNSILK & DANDELION TEA ——

This simple diuretic herbal remedy can help cut down excess fluid in the system. Dandelion leaves are rich in potassium while cornsilk is soothing for the urinary tract.

~ INGREDIENTS ~
50 g dried dandelion leaves (*Taraxacum officinale*)
30 g dried cornsilk (*Zea mays*)
20 g dried couchgrass rhizome (*Agropyron repens*)
water

~ HOW TO MAKE THE TEA ~
1 Mix the herbs and store in an airtight jar.

2 Place 2 teaspoons of the mixture in a tisane cup or small teapot. Add a cup of freshly boiled water and infuse for 10 minutes. Strain.

DOSAGE *Drink a cup 2 or 3 times a day while symptoms persist.*

CAUTION
• *Protein in the urine can be an indication that toxaemia is developing – other symptoms include headaches and raised blood pressure. If swelling in the ankles is not relieved by rest or is "pitting" (finger pressure leaves significant indentations in the flesh) seek professional medical help urgently.*

Preparing for childbirth

For centuries, women have taken herbs to prepare for an easy delivery, to ease labour pains and, ultimately, to help clear the placenta. Today modern medicine provides a battery of more sophisticated options but, for uncomplicated births, herbs still have an important role. About six weeks before the baby is due, start preparing with a daily cup of raspberry leaf tea (to make, see p. 64). Once labour starts, take Wood Betony & Rose Petal Tea.

—— WOOD BETONY & ROSE PETAL TEA ——

Wood betony helps to soothe the nervous system and ease tensions as well as stimulate uterine contractions. Rose petals are very uplifting – both physically and spiritually.

~ INGREDIENTS ~
50 g dried wood betony (*Stachys betonica*)
20 g dried rose petals (*Rosa gallica* or *R. centifolia*)
20 g dried raspberry leaves (*Rubus idaeus*)
10 g cinnamon stick (*Cinnamomum zeylanicum*)
500 ml water

~ HOW TO MAKE THE TEA ~
1. Mix the herbs and store in an airtight, pottery jar.

2. Put one-third into a teapot and pour on the freshly boiled water. Infuse for 10 minutes. Strain.

DOSAGE *Sip a mugful during labour. Repeat as often as required.*

Note: For the final stages of labour, add 10 g dried basil leaves to the herbal mixture and infuse as before.

Supplementary treatments
■ Once labour starts, massage the abdomen regularly with 10 drops each of clove and sage oil and 3 drops of rose oil in 10 ml of sweet almond oil.
■ Place a hot compress soaked in pot marigold infusion to which 2–3 drops of sage oil have been added, across the lower abdomen above the pubic area. Replace as the compress cools. (To make the compress, see p. 71).
■ Take homeopathic *Arnica* 6x tablets every 15–20 minutes after the birth for 2–4 hours to encourage recovery.

OTHER PROBLEMS IN PREGNANCY
See also: anaemia p. 109; backache p. 114; constipation p. 104; cramp p. 116; cystitis p. 127; haemorrhoids (piles) p. 106; high blood pressure p. 108; indigestion & heartburn p. 107; insomnia p. 113; vaginal infections p. 124; varicose veins p. 109.

Breastfeeding problems

Most child care experts acknowledge that "breast is best" for feeding a newborn baby, but establishing a relaxed pattern of breastfeeding can be difficult for many new mothers.

1. Increasing milk flow

Herbs can be used to encourage milk flow, and frequent feeds are also important. Mix together 20 g fennel seeds, 30 g dried goat's rue, 30 g dried vervain, 20 g dried nettles and a teaspoon of powdered cinnamon. Store the mix in an airtight dark glass or pottery jar. Take a single cup infusion (to make, see p. 64) 4 times a day. In addition, take 5 drops of chaste-tree berry tincture in warm water before breakfast. Avoid eating spicy food as the flavour may permeate the milk supply.

2. Sore nipples

Cracked and sore nipples can be a deterrent to breastfeeding and can lead to engorgement. Apply calendula cream (available over the counter) or a little runny honey mixed with sweet almond oil to the nipples at frequent intervals.

3. Engorgement & mastitis

If milk remains in the breast at the end of feeds they may become engorged and painful; if ducts become blocked, inflammation and infection – mastitis – may follow. A simple, but effective, herbal remedy for engorgement and mastitis is to place a cabbage leaf in the bra that has been washed thoroughly and softened by beating with a cooking mallet.

GENERAL CAUTIONS FOR PREGNANCY
• *Do not take alcoholic tinctures or tonic wines during pregnancy.*
• *Many herbs should be avoided in pregnancy. If in doubt, take professional advice. In the first 3 months avoid all medication and do not use the following herbs throughout pregnancy: arbor vitae, barberry, basil oil, black cohosh, blue cohosh, chamomile oil, Dang Gui, feverfew, goldenseal, greater celandine, juniper, lady's mantle, mistletoe, motherwort, mugwort, myrrh, pennyroyal, pokeroot, rue, shepherd's purse, southernwood, tansy and wormwood. Do not take therapeutic doses of the following during pregnancy: angelica, bitter orange, cayenne, celery seed, cinnamon, cowslip, elder bark, fennel, fenugreek, ginseng, lavender, marjoram, nutmeg, parsley, rhubarb root, senna, sage, tea, thyme, vervain, wild yam, wood betony and yarrow.*

URINARY TRACT PROBLEMS

REPEATED URINARY TRACT problems can be a sign of energy weakness or immune deficiency. Recurrent cystitis, for example, can be related to thrush, which often arises when the immune system is under stress. In Chinese medicine, kidney energy is linked to reproduction and creativity, and can be easily worn down by childbearing or over-work, leading to urinary problems. Some herbs are useful urinary antiseptics and help to clear infections, while others are warming and energizing, helping the system heal itself.

Cystitis

Cystitis is inflammation of the bladder and tends to be more common in women. The symptoms usually include cloudy, unpleasant-smelling urine, frequent urination, a burning sensation on passing water and low groin pain. It can be a recurrent problem, and may be triggered by bacteria passing into the urinary tract from faecal material or during intercourse.

— MARSHMALLOW & CORNSILK MIXTURE —
Marshmallow is rich in mucilages to ease inflamed membranes, while yarrow is astringent and healing.

~ INGREDIENTS ~
30 ml marshmallow tincture (*Althaea officinalis*)
30 ml bearberry tincture (*Arctostaphylos uva-ursi*)
20 ml cornsilk tincture (*Zea mays*)
10 ml couchgrass tincture (*Agropyron repens*)
10 ml yarrow tincture (*Achillea millefolium*)

~ HOW TO MAKE THE MIXTURE ~
To make the individual tinctures, see p. 68. Mix the tinctures together in a 100 ml sterilized, dark glass bottle.

DOSAGE *Put 5 ml in a tumbler and pour on half a glass of boiling water. Allow to cool, then sip. Take 4 times a day.*

CAUTION
• *Seek professional help if symptoms do not ease after a few days or if there are signs of kidney involvement (fever and loin pain).*

Supplementary treatments
■ Take the tea recommended for urethritis on p. 118.
■ Take 2 x 200 mg capsules of echinacea 3 times a day to fight infections. Drink plenty of water and avoid alcohol.

CAUTION FOR KIDNEY PROBLEMS
• *Kidney infections require professional treatment. Seek medical help if a bladder or urinary tract infection is accompanied by loin pain or feverishness. Kidney stones should always be referred to a professional practitioner.*

Urinary stones

Urinary stones are formed from deposits of uric acid or calcium salts crystallizing in highly concentrated urine and collecting in the urinary tract. The urine usually appears cloudy and passing water may feel uncomfortable and "gritty".

—— PELLITORY & GRAVELROOT TEA ——
Both pellitory-of-the-wall and gravelroot are effective at breaking up and encouraging elimination of urinary stones. Pellitory is a Mediterranean relative of the stinging nettle, while gravelroot originates from the USA.

~ INGREDIENTS ~
15 g dried gravelroot (*Eupatorium purpureum*)
10 g dried marshmallow root (*Althaea officinalis*)
750 ml water
10 g dried pellitory-of-the-wall (*Parietaria diffusa*)
10 g celery seed (*Apium graveolens*)
5 g dried cornsilk (*Zea mays*)

~ HOW TO MAKE THE TEA ~
1 Put the gravelroot, marshmallow and water in a pan and simmer for 15–20 minutes to make a decoction.

2 Place the other herbs in a teapot or jug and pour the simmering decoction over them. Infuse for 10 minutes. Strain into a jug. Cover and store in a cool place.

DOSAGE *Drink a large mugful 4 times a day.*

CHILDREN'S COMPLAINTS

MANY CHILDREN'S AILMENTS are self-limiting and mild, although symptoms can be dramatic, with sudden fevers and soaring temperatures. Home treatment is often sufficient, but it is important to seek medical help urgently if symptoms are acute or of increasing severity. Herbs provide gentle remedies that are safe even for young babies.

CAUTION

Some remedies can taste bitter and may need to be sweetened with fruit juice or honey. Only give children under a year pasteurized honey or honey that has been boiled for 5 minutes.

DOSAGE FOR BABIES & CHILDREN

All doses in this section are suitable for babies and children. When giving other remedies to children, remember to reduce the adult dose. For children under 2 years give a fifth of the adult dose increasing gradually to reach a quarter at 3 or 4 (depending on the size of the child), a third at 6 or 7, a half at 8 or 9, and then increasing to the full adult dose at puberty.

Babies: Sleeplessness

Sleepless babies soon make the rest of the household tense and irritable, compounding the problem. Make sure the room is not too hot, the baby is comfortable, feels safe and secure, and is not hungry or thirsty. Give lots of cuddles.

CHAMOMILE BATH

Chamomile is one of the best herbs for small babies – sedative and calming for the digestive system, it is ideal for soothing over-excitement which can contribute to sleeplessness.

~ INGREDIENTS ~
2 drops chamomile oil (*Matricaria recutita*)
1 drop lavender oil (*Lavandula angustifolia*)

~ HOW TO USE THE MIXTURE ~
Add the oils to the bath and agitate the water well before bathing the baby.

Supplementary treatments
■ Gentle massage can help calm small babies – stroke arms repeatedly rather than trying body massage. Use a single drop of chamomile oil in 20 ml of sweet almond oil.
■ Avoid caffeine if breastfeeding. If the child is taking solids, check foods for artificial colourants or additives and ensure adequate intake of vitamins and minerals.
■ Give 25–50 ml infusion at night (to make, see p. 64) using 10 g of dried chamomile flowers, catmint, wood betony or lemon balm to 500 ml water.

Babies: Nappy rash

Nappy rash is a common affliction and can be very painful and irritating. It can be caused by irregular or inefficient nappy changes and it can also be related to digestive problems and yeast infections, so it is important to check the diet of the baby (or the mother if breastfeeding) and eliminate likely irritants.

COMFREY & TEA TREE OIL

Comfrey increases the rate of cell growth thereby speeding repair of damaged tissue. Protective, waterproof ointments or infused oils should be used for nappy rash rather than creams, which soften the skin still further. Tea tree oil is added to counter infection.

~ INGREDIENTS ~
250 g dried comfrey leaf (*Symphytum officinale*)
500 ml sunflower oil
10 ml tea tree oil (*Melaleuca alternifolia*)

~ HOW TO MAKE THE OIL ~

1 Make a hot infused oil using the comfrey and sunflower oil. For instructions, see p. 72.

2 Add the tea tree oil to the infused oil and mix well. Store in sterilized, dark glass bottles.

APPLICATION *At each nappy change, make sure the baby is well cleaned and dried (using a hairdryer on a cool setting if necessary). Gently apply a little of the oil to the affected area. Leave the nappy off for as long as possible.*

Babies: Colic

The gut spasms and discomfort of colic can often be caused by rushed or tense feeding times. Check the baby's diet (or the mother's diet, if breastfeeding) to eliminate likely irritants such as hot spices, cow's milk or wheat, and ensure that both mother and baby are relaxed and calm at meal times.

—— CATMINT TEA ——

Catmint is an ideal remedy for children – gentle and soothing. It both eases gut spasms and acts as a mild sedative encouraging sleep.

~ INGREDIENTS ~

10 g dried catmint (*Nepeta cataria*)
175 ml water

~ HOW TO MAKE THE TEA ~

Place the catmint in a teapot. Add freshly boiled water and infuse for 10 minutes. Strain. The surplus can be stored in a cool place in a covered jug for up to 48 hours.

DOSAGE *Give 25–50 ml of the warm infusion before meals, reheating each dose.*

Supplementary treatments

■ If breastfeeding, and tension is a problem, mothers should drink an infusion of skullcap, vervain, wood betony or chamomile tea before feeds (to make, see p. 64).
■ Soak a compress (to make, see p. 71) in an infusion made from 15 g chamomile flowers and 500 ml water (to make, see p. 64) and apply to the baby's abdomen to relieve colicky pains.

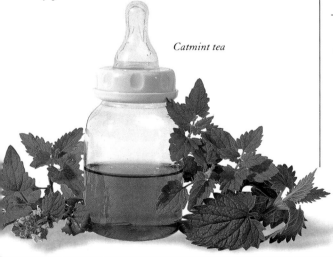

Catmint tea

Babies: Teething

Teething pains can be a problem for babies from the age of four months (or younger in some cases).

—— CHAMOMILE & SAGE GUM RUB ——

Chamomile oil acts as a soothing sedative while sage oil is astringent, healing and antiseptic, helping to soothe sore gums.

~ INGREDIENTS ~

4 drops chamomile oil (*Matricaria recutita*)
2 drops sage oil (*Salvia officinalis*)
2 drops rosemary oil (*Rosmarinus officinalis*)
20 ml sunflower or sweet almond oil

~ HOW TO MAKE THE RUB ~

Pour the oils into a 50 ml sterilized, dark glass bottle and shake well.

APPLICATION *Smear a small amount of the oil on your finger and gently rub the baby's gums with it. Repeat 3 or 4 times a day.*

Supplementary treatment

■ Give 25–50 ml of a weak infusion of sedative herbs such as linden flowers or chamomile before feeds (use 10 g dried herb to 500 ml water, to make, see p. 64).

Babies: Cradle cap

Cradle cap is a scaly dermatitis which can affect the scalps of small babies and can be caused by over-active sweat glands. It is not serious or contagious.

—— HEARTSEASE & MARIGOLD OIL ——

Heartsease is a soothing and anti-inflammatory herb, useful for a wide range of skin disorders. Pot marigold is antifungal and astringent, encouraging healing.

~ INGREDIENTS ~

100 g pot marigold petals (*Calendula officinalis*)
150 g heartsease (*Viola tricolor*)
750 ml sunflower oil

~ HOW TO MAKE THE OIL ~

Make a hot infused oil following the instructions on p. 73.

APPLICATION *Apply a little of the oil to the affected area several times a day. Massage very gently, especially on newborn babies whose fontanelles (soft spots) have yet to close completely.*

Children: Hyperactivity

Symptoms of hyperactivity include sleeplessness, poor attention span, tearfulness and aggressive behaviour. Food intolerance or pollution are often to blame, or the child may be suffering from emotional difficulties. The diet should contain an adequate supply of B vitamins, zinc and iron (found in cereals, meat and many vegetables). Avoid all artificial colourings, preservatives and additives, and strictly control intake of sugar, chocolate, milk and caffeine.

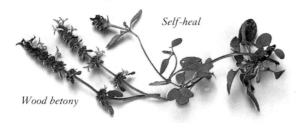

Self-heal

Wood betony

—— SELF-HEAL & WOOD BETONY TEA ——

Self-heal is a common garden weed, used as a wound herb in the West. The Chinese regard it as cooling and cleansing for the liver, where pollutants and food additives tend to accumulate. Wood betony has a sedative action.

~ INGREDIENTS ~
10 g dried self-heal spikes
(*Xia Ku Cao – Prunella vulgaris*)
5 g dried wood betony (*Stachys betonica*)
5 g dried borage (*Borago officinalis*)
500 ml water
2–3 drops liquorice fluid extract (*Glycyrrhiza glabra*)
or peppermint emulsion (*Mentha piperita*) per dose

~ HOW TO MAKE THE TEA ~
Place the dried herbs in a teapot and add freshly boiled water. Infuse for 10 minutes and strain. The surplus can be stored in a covered jug in a cool place for up to 48 hours.

DOSAGE *Give a 100–150 ml dose for 3–6-year-olds 3 times a day. Flavour with liquorice extract or peppermint emulsion as required (available over the counter).*

Supplementary treatments
■ Evening primrose oil can help – give 250–500 mg daily. Zinc supplements can also be useful. Give 10–20 mg daily.
■ If environmental pollution is a problem give kelp supplements, which help cleanse heavy metals from the system. Give 10–20 mg daily.

Children: Bedwetting

Regular bedwetting in young children can be the result of urinary infections, dietary deficiencies, minor physical problems with the urinary tract or emotional upsets. Take professional advice to identify the cause.

—— CORNSILK & ST JOHN'S WORT TEA ——

Cornsilk is soothing and healing for the urinary tract. St John's wort is useful for anxiety and nervous tension.

~ INGREDIENTS ~
5 g dried cornsilk (*Zea mays*)
10 g dried St John's wort (*Hypericum perforatum*)
500 ml water

~ HOW TO MAKE THE TEA ~
Place the dried herbs in a teapot and add freshly boiled water. Infuse for 10 minutes and strain. The surplus can be stored in a covered jug in a cool place for up to 48 hours.

DOSAGE *Give 4-year-olds a 100 ml dose 3 times a day. Increase the quantity to 150 ml for 8-year-olds.*

Supplementary treatment
■ Sweet sumach tincture is a traditional remedy for bedwetting. For 4–8-year-olds, give 5–10 drops in a little warm water 3 times a day (to make, see p. 68).

Children: Nits

Nits are the eggs of head lice. They spread quickly, and outbreaks in schools are commonplace. Suspect infection if children persistently scratch their heads.

—— TEA TREE RINSE ——

Tea tree oil is extracted from an Australian tree and is one of the most antiseptic and antibacterial herbs available. Unlike many oils, it does not irritate the skin.

~ INGREDIENTS ~
5 ml tea tree oil (*Melaleuca alternifolia*)
1 ml lemon oil (*Citrus limon*)
500 ml warm water

~ HOW TO MAKE THE RINSE ~
Mix the oils in a bottle and add the water. Shake well.

APPLICATION *Use as a final rinse after shampooing. Repeat each day until the infection clears.*

Children: Threadworms

Threadworms are common in children and are highly contagious, so scrupulous hygiene is essential for the whole family. Worms lay eggs in the anus at night, so examine the child's bottom before bedtime and remove worms where possible. Worms have a life-cycle of two weeks, so treatment should be repeated after a fortnight to eliminate the problem completely.

—— CARROT & WORMWOOD MIXTURE ——

Carrot is toxic for threadworms, and in some folk traditions the child would be fed nothing but raw, grated carrot for two days to clear the problem. Wormwood also clears threadworms from the system. It has an extremely bitter taste and fennel is added to make it more palatable.

~ INGREDIENTS ~

60 ml carrot juice
10 drops wormwood tincture (*Artemisia absinthium*)
20 drops fennel tincture (*Foeniculum officinalis*)

~ HOW TO MAKE THE MIXTURE ~

Carrot juice is available commercially, or can be made using a food processor or juicer. To make the tinctures, see p. 68. Stir the tinctures into the juice. This quantity is sufficient for a single dose.

DOSAGE *Give a dose each morning before breakfast for 4 days. Repeat 2 weeks later.*

Supplementary treatments

■ Garlic is effective at clearing worms. Give 2 x 200 mg garlic capsules each morning or finely chop a clove and mix with a little honey stirred into a cup of warm milk.
■ Cabbage is another effective remedy. Juice fresh leaves in a food processor or juicer and use 60 ml as an alternative to carrot juice in the Carrot & Wormwood Mixture.

Children: Croup

Croup usually affects children aged between about six months and two years. It is caused by inflammation and obstruction of the larynx. Viral infections in the respiratory tract are generally to blame and the barking cough that results can sound quite frightening.

— LAVENDER & EUCALYPTUS STEAMER & RUB —

A damp, steamy atmosphere can rapidly ease symptoms. Lavender and eucalyptus oils are antiseptic and healing.

~ INGREDIENTS ~

20 drops lavender oil (*Lavandula angustifolia*)
10 drops eucalyptus oil (*Eucalyptus globulus*)
10 drops pine oil (*Pinus sylvestris*)
25 ml sweet almond or wheatgerm oil

~ HOW TO APPLY THE STEAMER & RUB ~

1 Combine 10 drops of lavender, 5 drops of eucalyptus and 5 drops of pine oil. Add to a bath of steaming water and sit the child close by until symptoms ease (do not put the child in the bath).

2 Add the same combination of oils (20 drops total) to the sweet almond or wheatgerm oil and massage a little into the child's chest after the steam treatment.

CAUTION
• *Croup can be a symptom of more severe respiratory problems. Seek professional help if symptoms persist for more than 2 or 3 days or appear to be getting worse.*

Supplementary treatments
■ Give tinctures of wild cherry and white horehound (up to 5 drops of each) in a little warm water 3 times a day. To make the tinctures, see p. 68.
■ Use a humidifier in the child's room at night.

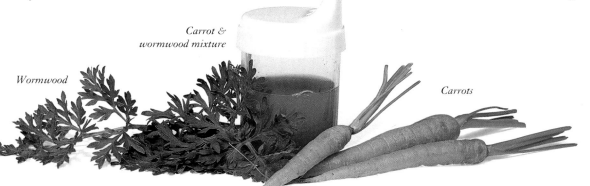

Carrot & wormwood mixture

Wormwood

Carrots

Children: Mumps

Mumps is a viral disease, affecting various glands. In children, these are generally the salivary glands in the throat, and the condition is usually mild and suitable for home treatment. Adolescents and adults, however, should seek professional treatment, as the condition is potentially more serious, often affecting the testes.

THYME & SAGE GARGLE

Antiseptic gargles and mouthwashes can help combat the symptoms of mumps. Both thyme and sage are effective herbs – use either, or, as here, a mixture of the two.

~ INGREDIENTS ~
15 g dried thyme (*Thymus vulgaris*)
15 g dried sage (*Salvia officinalis*)
500 ml water

~ HOW TO MAKE THE GARGLE ~

1. Place the dried herbs in a teapot and and add freshly boiled water.

2. Infuse for 15 minutes and strain. The surplus may be stored in a covered jug in a cool place or refrigerator for up to 48 hours.

DOSAGE *Use 50 ml of the infusion diluted with 50 ml of hot water as a gargle, repeating the treatment every 1–2 hours while symptoms are severe.*

Supplementary treatments
■ Follow the recommendations for fevers given on p. 87.
■ Mix 50 ml cleavers tincture and 25 ml each of echinacea and marigold tincture and give in 5 ml doses in warm water 3 times a day to counter infections and cleanse the lymphatic system. To make the tinctures, see p. 68.

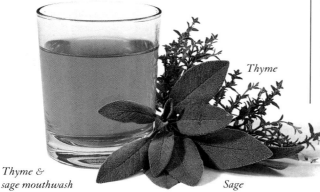

Thyme

*Thyme &
sage mouthwash*   *Sage*

Children: Chickenpox

In children, chickenpox is usually a mild, if highly contagious, infection. In adults, the same virus can produce shingles. Chickenpox is characterized by rashes, which soon turn into a crop of spots that blister and lead to scabs. The rashes are generally accompanied by a mild fever. Spots are most common on the scalp, face and body and are very irritating. Scratching the scabs can lead to scars.

BORAGE & CHICKWEED LOTION

Chickweed can be used for a variety of irritant skin conditions, including eczema. Although it is often used as a cream, in this mixture it is combined with borage juice, which can also help to reduce skin irritation, to form a cooling lotion.

~ INGREDIENTS ~
10 g dried, or 30 g fresh chickweed (*Stellaria media*)
100 ml water
30 ml borage juice (*Borago officinalis*)
25 ml distilled witch hazel (*Hamamelis virginiana*)

~ HOW TO MAKE THE LOTION ~

1. Place the chickweed in a teapot and add the freshly boiled water. Infuse for 15 minutes and strain.

2. Mix 45 ml of the chickweed infusion with the borage juice (available over the counter) and witch hazel in a 100 ml dark glass bottle. Shake well.

APPLICATION *Soak a cottonwool pad in the mixture and apply gently to the chickenpox rash, taking care not to damage the scabs. Repeat as often as necessary to soothe the irritation.*

Supplementary treatments
■ Give a cup of standard infusion of skullcap, wood betony or chamomile 2–3 times daily as a general relaxant to calm the child (to make the infusion, see p. 64).
■ If fever is a problem, follow the recommendations given on p. 87.
■ Give 3 x 200 mg echinacea capsules or 5 ml echinacea tincture in a little warm water 3 times a day before meals. To make the capsules and tincture, see pp. 70 and 68.

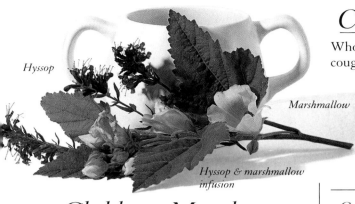

Hyssop

Marshmallow

Hyssop & marshmallow infusion

Children: Whooping cough

Whooping cough often starts slowly with a mild cough and cold. Production of sticky mucus soon follows, with breathlessness, a convulsive and distressing cough, and a tendency to vomit.

CAUTION
- *Before the age of three, whooping cough can be a dangerous illness. Seek professional help in all cases.*

— WILD LETTUCE & THYME TEA —
Coughing spasms can be painful and exhausting. The sedative effect of wild lettuce helps to calm the child, while thyme is antiseptic and combines with other expectorants in the mix to help clear mucus. This tea can form a useful adjunct to professional treatments.

~ INGREDIENTS ~
5 g dried elecampane root (*Inula helenium*)
5 g liquorice root (*Glycyrrhiza glabra*)
750 ml water
10 g dried wild lettuce (*Lactuca virosa*)
5 g dried thyme (*Thymus vulgaris*)
10 g dried mullein flowers (*Verbascum thapsus*)

~ HOW TO MAKE THE TEA ~
1 Put the elecampane, liquorice and water in a pan and simmer for 20 minutes to make a decoction.

2 Mix the remaining dried herbs in a teapot and pour on the simmering decoction. Infuse for 10 minutes and strain.

DOSAGE *Give a large mugful up to 6 times a day.*

Supplementary treatments
■ Ensure the child's room is well ventilated and dry.
■ Mix 2 ml each of hyssop, cypress and basil oil in 50 ml of sweet almond oil. Rub on to the child's chest 2 or 3 times a day. Alternatively, put the undiluted essential oils into a vaporizer or diffuser in the child's room at night.
■ Give 3 x 200 mg echinacea capsules twice a day if the child can swallow them. If not, give 5 ml echinacea tincture in warm water twice daily. To make, see pp. 70 and 68.

— Other Childhood Ailments —
See also the following ailments in the adult section: constipation p. 104; diarrhoea p. 105; earache p. 91; gastritis p. 106 and nausea & vomiting p. 107.
Note: See p. 128 for advice on reducing adult dosages to suit children.

Children: Measles

Measles is a highly contagious viral disease, characterized by a heavy cold, harsh, dry cough, a blotchy rash that usually starts behind the ears, and bloodshot, light-sensitive eyes. It usually occurs in local epidemics and complications include pneumonia and middle-ear infections. In many cases it is important to seek professional help.

— HYSSOP & MARSHMALLOW INFUSION —
Relaxing expectorants help to soothe the coughing associated with measles. Hyssop is an ideal expectorant for children and marshmallow is a demulcent, helping to lubricate the mucous membranes.

~ INGREDIENTS ~
30 g dried hyssop (*Hyssopus officinalis*)
30 g dried marshmallow leaf (*Althaea officinalis*)
30 g dried ribwort plantain (*Plantago major*)
water
2 ml liquorice fluid extract per dose (*Glycyrrhiza glabra*)

~ HOW TO MAKE THE INFUSION ~
Mix the herbs and store in an airtight container. Place a teaspoon of the mixture in a tisane cup or small teapot and add freshly boiled water. Infuse for 10 minutes and strain.

DOSAGE *Give a teacup dose 4 times a day, before meals and at night, adding the liquorice fluid extract as a flavouring.*

Supplementary treatments
■ Follow the recommendations for fever on p. 87.
■ Give 3 x 200 mg echinacea capsules or 5 ml echinacea tincture 3 times daily. To make, see pp. 70 and 68.
■ Use well-strained eyebright or self-heal infusions in an eyebath to soothe irritation. See p. 79.

HEDGEROW HEALERS

"ALL NATURE," WROTE the sixteenth-century herbalist Paracelsus, "is like one single apothecary's shop, covered only with the roof of heaven. . . ". In an emergency outdoors, wild plants can provide help until more conventional remedies are available. However, as Paracelsus also pointed out, "In all things there is a poison and there is nothing without poison – it depends only upon the dose whether a poison is poison or not. . . ". Some healing plants have a nastier side to them and careful handling is required – especially if small children are around.

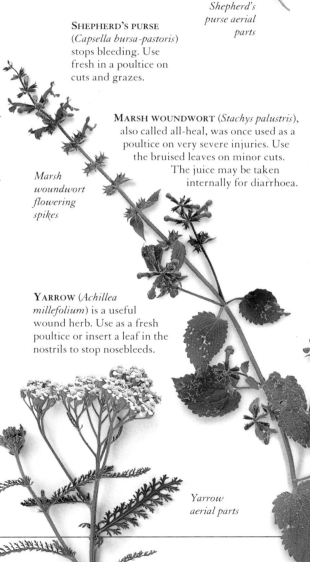

Shepherd's purse aerial parts

Wild herbs

The following may be gathered for use in home-made remedies, and many of them are useful in emergency first aid – when minor accidents happen on country walks and the first aid box is out of reach.

SHEPHERD'S PURSE (*Capsella bursa-pastoris*) stops bleeding. Use fresh in a poultice on cuts and grazes.

─────── CAUTIONS ───────
- *Use a botanical field guide to identify plants correctly.*
- *The remedies listed here are for emergency use or for minor problems. Seek medical help for serious cuts, burns and sprains as soon as possible – an anti-tetanus injection may be recommended.*

MARSH WOUNDWORT (*Stachys palustris*), also called all-heal, was once used as a poultice on very severe injuries. Use the bruised leaves on minor cuts. The juice may be taken internally for diarrhoea.

Marsh woundwort flowering spikes

BEAR'S BREECHES (*Acanthus mollis*) Apply the crushed leaves to minor burns and scalds.
COMMON MALLOW (*Malva sylvestris*) The leaves and flowers can be used as a poultice for wounds.
CORNFLOWER (*Centaurea cyanus*) Bathe sore eyes with a well-strained infusion.
CREEPING JENNY (*Lysimachia nummularia*) A poultice of fresh leaves or a compress made from a strong infusion can be used to treat wounds and sores.
HERB BENNET (*Geum urbanum*) Chew the clove-flavoured root to sweeten the breath. A decoction can ease chills and diarrhoea.
JACK-BY-THE-HEDGE (*Alliaria petiolata*) Also known as garlic mustard; the fresh leaves can be crushed and applied to insect bites to relieve itching.

MEADOWSWEET (*Filipendula ulmaria*) Commonly found in wayside ditches; use the infusion to settle stomach upsets.
PURPLE LOOSESTRIFE (*Lythrum salicaria*) The infusion may be taken for diarrhoea or used in compresses to help ease skin rashes.
STINGING NETTLE (*Urtica dioica*) Use the infusion in compresses for eczema, as a gargle for sore throats and mouth ulcers, or on cottonwool plugs to stop nosebleeds.
TOADFLAX (*Linaria vulgaris*) Make a poultice with fresh leaves to treat cuts or piles. A well-strained infusion can be an effective eye wash for sore eyes.
WHITE DEADNETTLE (*Lamium album*) The infusion may be taken internally for cystitis or used in a compress to treat piles.

YARROW (*Achillea millefolium*) is a useful wound herb. Use as a fresh poultice or insert a leaf in the nostrils to stop nosebleeds.

Yarrow aerial parts

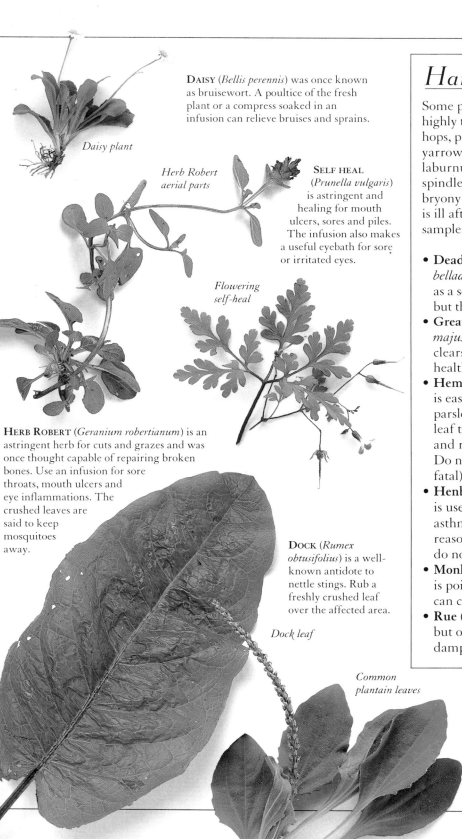

DAISY (*Bellis perennis*) was once known as bruisewort. A poultice of the fresh plant or a compress soaked in an infusion can relieve bruises and sprains.

Daisy plant

Herb Robert aerial parts

SELF HEAL (*Prunella vulgaris*) is astringent and healing for mouth ulcers, sores and piles. The infusion also makes a useful eyebath for sore or irritated eyes.

Flowering self-heal

HERB ROBERT (*Geranium robertianum*) is an astringent herb for cuts and grazes and was once thought capable of repairing broken bones. Use an infusion for sore throats, mouth ulcers and eye inflammations. The crushed leaves are said to keep mosquitoes away.

DOCK (*Rumex obtusifolius*) is a well-known antidote to nettle stings. Rub a freshly crushed leaf over the affected area.

Dock leaf

Common plantain leaves

COMMON PLANTAIN (*Plantago major*) makes a readily available remedy for insect bites and stings. Rub the fresh leaves on to the affected part.

Handle with care

Some plants and flowers are highly toxic. Borage, chamomile, hops, primulas, runner beans and yarrow can cause rashes. Holly, laburnum, mistletoe, privet, spindle, sweet pea and white bryony have toxic fruits. If a child is ill after eating a plant, take a sample with you to the hospital.

- **Deadly nightshade** (*Atropa belladonna*) is used by herbalists as a sedative and antispasmodic, but the black berries are fatal.
- **Greater celandine** (*Chelidonium majus*) has a yellow sap that clears warts, but can irritate healthy skin. Handle with care.
- **Hemlock** (*Conium maculatum*) is easily mistaken for cow parsley or sweet cicely: look for leaf textures, smell, seed shapes and red blotches on the stem. Do not swallow (this can be fatal); handle with care.
- **Henbane** (*Hyoscyamus niger*) is used medicinally to treat asthma and colic. It is reasonably safe to handle, but do not swallow the fresh plant.
- **Monkshood** (*Aconitum napellus*) is poisonous and touching it can cause numbness.
- **Rue** (*Ruta graveolens*) is edible, but on sunny days, sap and damp leaves can cause a rash.

THE HERBAL FIRST AID BOX

MOST HOUSEHOLDS HAVE their regular stock of over-the-counter pharmaceuticals for emergencies, but herbal alternatives can be just as effective, often offering more healing properties from a small number of basic ingredients. The kitchen cupboard can also be useful, providing garlic, ginger, tea, honey and other ingredients. Supplement these household items with over-the-counter herbal preparations.

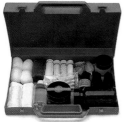

FIRST AID BOX
Keep the first aid box easily accessible, but out of the reach of children.

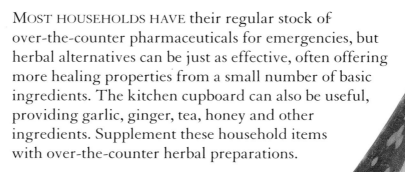

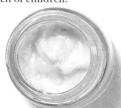

ARNICA CREAM
Effective for bruises and sprains. Do not use on broken skin.

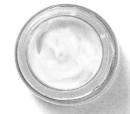

CHICKWEED CREAM
Valuable for drawing splinters, boils and insect stings or for easing burns, scalds and eczema.

ALOE VERA
To soothe minor burns, scalds or sunburn, break off a leaf from an aloe plant, split it open and apply the thick gel to the affected area.

TEA TREE OIL
One of the most antiseptic and antifungal oils; use for cuts and grazes as well as on warts and cold sores.

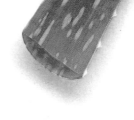

MARIGOLD CREAM
Often sold as calendula; an antiseptic and antifungal cream, used for cuts, grazes and dry skin.

GARLIC
Rub fresh cloves on acne and other infected spots. Use crushed garlic to draw corns. Take internally for chest infections and thrush.

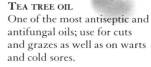

HOMEOPATHIC ARNICA 6X
Essential for domestic shocks or accidents, one tablet should be taken at 30 minute intervals until the patient feels calmer and more settled.

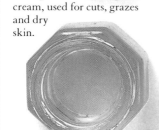

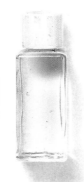

DISTILLED WITCH HAZEL
Use for minor burns and sunburn. Soak a swab in witch hazel to staunch wounds. Frozen witch hazel soothes insect bites, varicose veins and bruises. Keep a clearly labelled icecube tray of witch hazel in the freezer.

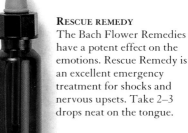

RESCUE REMEDY
The Bach Flower Remedies have a potent effect on the emotions. Rescue Remedy is an excellent emergency treatment for shocks and nervous upsets. Take 2–3 drops neat on the tongue.

HONEY
Draws pus and poisons out of wounds. Useful for colds, mixed with hot lemon juice and water.

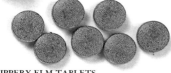

EVENING PRIMROSE OIL
A useful hangover cure, restoring liver function. Take a large dose (2–3 g) "the morning after" for rapid relief.

LAVENDER OIL
Dilute 2–3 drops in a teaspoon of sweet almond oil and use to massage the temples and neck for tension headaches and migraine. Use the same mix for burns and scalds.

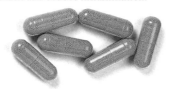

SLIPPERY ELM TABLETS
Take 1–2 x 200 g capsules for indigestion, gastritis and stomach upsets, to line the stomach and reduce inflammation.

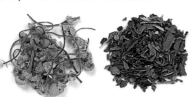

ECHINACEA CAPSULES
A valuable standby for colds and flu. Take 2 x 200 g capsules or tablets 3 times a day at the first hint of infection.

Chamomile   *Peppermint*

DRIED HERBS
Keep an assortment of dried herbs or herbal teabags handy for infusions. Use chamomile flowers for shock, nervous upsets, insomnia or indigestion; fennel or peppermint for indigestion; lavender for headaches and migraines; vervain for stress and digestive problems and elderflower for catarrh.

Herbs for holidays

Holidays can be easily spoiled by minor ailments. Basic hygiene rules are essential in exotic locations: peel fruit and do not eat any other raw foods, and do not drink tapwater or have icecubes in drinks. If stomach upsets and diarrhoea occur, try eating papaya – a traditional remedy in many tropical areas – or drink strong black tea without milk or sugar. Take a holiday first aid kit to cope with other problems.

FIRST AID CHECKLIST

• Cuts and grazes: tea tree oil or pot marigold cream. Dab a little on to the affected part.
• Diarrhoea: mix equal amounts of bistort, honeysuckle and marshmallow tinctures. Take 5 ml in warm water every 2–3 hours.
• Heatstroke: sugar and salt. Take ½ a teaspoon of each in some water.
• Insect bites, cuts and grazes: use 2–3 drops of lemon balm oil in a teaspoon of sweet almond oil or St John's wort and marigold tinctures. Dab on to the affected part.
• Jet lag: Siberian ginseng or chamomile teabags.
• Shock: take a homeopathic *Arnica* 6x pill at 30 minute intervals.
• Sprains and bruises: arnica or comfrey cream (do not use on broken skin).
• Stomach upsets: meadowsweet tincture. Take 5 ml in warm water 3–4 times a day. Chamomile or peppermint teabags are also useful.
• Sunburn: 5 ml lavender oil combined with 20 ml infused St John's wort oil. Dab on the skin.
• Travel sickness and vomiting: crystallized ginger or ginger capsules.

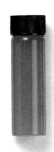 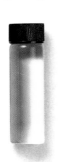 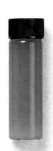 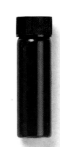 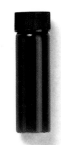

St John's wort & lavender oil   *Tea tree oil*   *St John's wort & marigold tincture*   *Meadowsweet tincture*   *Honeysuckle, bistort & marshmallow tincture*

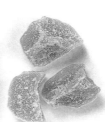 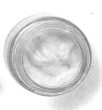 

Arnica 6x tablets   *Crystallized ginger*   *Arnica cream*   *Herbal teabags*

OTHER MEDICINAL HERBS

Each entry gives the common name, botanical name, parts used and their actions.
Caution: do not take essential oils internally except when directed to do so by a professional practitioner.

ANGELICA: *Angelica archangelica*
Leaves: carminative, antispasmodic, diaphoretic, expectorant, diuretic, digestive tonic, antirheumatic, uterine stimulant. **Caution:** avoid large doses in pregnancy and in diabetes.

ANISE: *Pimpinella anisum*
Essential oil, seeds: expectorant, carminative, antiseptic, antispasmodic.

ASHWAGANDHA: *Withania somnifera*
Root: tonic, aphrodisiac, sedative, astringent, nervine.

BAI SHAO, WHITE PAEONY:
Paeonia lactiflora
Root: antibacterial, reduces blood pressure, antispasmodic, anti-inflammatory, analgesic, tranquillizing.

BAI ZHI: *Atractylodes macrocephala*
Rhizome: energy tonic, carminative, diuretic.

BASIL: *Ocimum basilicum*
Leaves, essential oil: antidepressant, antiseptic, stimulating, soothing, prevents vomiting, carminative, febrifuge, tonic. **Caution:** avoid the essential oil in pregnancy.

BAYBERRY: *Myrica cerifera*
Bark: stimulant, astringent, diaphoretic.

BEARBERRY, UVA-URSI:
Arctostaphylos uva-ursi
Leaves: astringent, urinary antiseptic. **Caution:** high doses may cause nausea.

BENZOIN: *Styrax benzoin*
Essential oil, gum: expectorant, astringent, antispasmodic.

BISTORT: *Polygonum bistorta*
Root: astringent, anticatarrhal, styptic.

BLACK HAW: *Viburnum prunifolium*
Root, bark: antispasmodic, sedative, astringent, relaxant, tonic, uterine relaxant, anti-inflammatory.

BLACK HOREHOUND: *Ballota nigra*
Aerial parts: prevents vomiting, stimulant, tonic.

BLADDERWRACK *see* **KELP**

BLUE FLAG: *Iris versicolor*
Rhizome: anti-inflammatory, stimulant, diuretic.

BOGBEAN: *Menyanthes trifoliata*
Leaves: antirheumatic, bitter, tonic.

BOLDO: *Peumus boldo*
Leaves: liver stimulant, diuretic.

BONESET: *Eupatorium perfoliatum*
Aerial parts: diaphoretic, laxative, antispasmodic, expectorant.
Caution: high doses can cause vomiting.

BORAGE: *Borago officinalis*
Leaves, flowers: adrenal stimulants, diuretic, promote lactation, febrifuge, antirheumatic, diaphoretic, expectorant. **Seed oil:** a source of gamma-linolenic acid.
Note: restricted herb in Australia and New Zealand.

BUCKWHEAT:
Fagopyrum esculentum
Leaves: reduce blood pressure, repair blood vessels.

BU GU ZHI: *Psoralea corylifolia*
Fruit: diuretic, astringent, antibacterial, kidney tonic.
Caution: can cause photosensitivity of the skin.

CABBAGE: *Brassica oleracea*
Leaves: anti-inflammatory, anti-bacterial, liver decongestant.

CAJEPUT: *Melaleuca leucadendra*
Essential oil: diaphoretic, expectorant, aromatic.

CAMPHOR: *Cinnamomum camphora*
Gum oil: carminative, analgesic, antiseptic, sedative, stimulant.
Caution: do not take internally.

CARAWAY: *carum carvi*
Seeds: digestive stimulant, antiseptic.

CASCARA: *Rhamnus purshiana*
Bark: digestive tonic, laxative.
Caution: avoid in pregnancy.

CATMINT: *Nepeta cataria*
Aerial parts: antispasmodic,

carminative, digestive stimulant, diaphoretic.

CHASTE-TREE: *Vitex agnus-castus*
Berries: hormone stimulant.
Caution: high doses may cause formication (a sensation of ants crawling on the skin).

CHICKWEED: *Stellaria media*
Aerial parts: astringent, antirheumatic, heals wounds, demulcent.

CHINESE CHRYSANTHEMUM *see*
JU HUA

CLARY: *Salvia sclarea*
Essential oil: carminative, nerve tonic, uterine stimulant.
Cautions: high doses are toxic and may cause headaches. Avoid in pregnancy.

CLOVE: *Syzygium aromaticum*
Essential oil, flower buds: carminative, antispasmodic, prevent vomiting. **Caution:** do not exceed stated dose.

COMFREY: *Symphytum officinale*
Aerial parts, root: cell proliferator, astringent, heals wounds, demulcent, expectorant.
Cautions: avoid excessive internal consumption of the herb. Use only on clean wounds.
Note: restricted herb in Australia and New Zealand.

COUCHGRASS: *Agropyron repens*
Rhizome: cleansing diuretic, demulcent.

COWSLIP: *Primula veris*
Flowers: sedative nervine, calming, astringent, promote sweating. **Root:** stimulating, expectorant, astringent, promotes sweating. **Cautions:** avoid in aspirin-sensitivity or if taking blood-thinning drugs. Do not take high doses in pregnancy.

CRANESBILL: *Geranium maculatum*
Leaves, root: astringent.

CRAMP BARK *see* **GUELDER ROSE**

CYPRESS: *Cupressus sempervirens*
Essential oil: antiseptic, sedative.

DAMIANA: *Turnera diffusa*
Aerial parts: aphrodisiac, diuretic, urinary antiseptic, laxative, nervine.

DANG SHEN: *Codonopsis pilosula*
Root: demulcent, expectorant, tonic.

DEVIL'S CLAW: *Harpagophytum procumbens*
Tuber: diuretic, anti-inflammatory, antirheumatic, analgesic, sedative, liver stimulant.

DILL: *Anethum graveolens*
Seeds: carminative.

ELECAMPANE: *Inula helenium*
Root, flowers: tonic, stimulating expectorant, diaphoretic, antibacterial, antifungal, antiparasitic, digestive stimulant.

EPHEDRA *see* **MA HUANG**

FALSE UNICORN ROOT, HELONIAS:
Chamaelirium luteum
Rhizome: diuretic, emetic, uterine tonic.

FENUGREEK: *Trigonella foenum-graecum*
Seeds: digestive tonic, anti-inflammatory, promote milk flow, locally demulcent, uterine stimulant, reduce blood sugar levels, aphrodisiac. **Aerial parts:** antispasmodic. **Cautions:** avoid in pregnancy. The aerial parts may be used in labour. Insulin-dependent diabetics should avoid unless under professional guidance.

FIGWORT: *Scrophularia nodosa*
Aerial parts: diuretic, laxative, heart stimulant, circulatory stimulant, anti-inflammatory.
Caution: avoid in cases of abnormally rapid heartbeat.

FORSYTHIA *see* **LIAN QIAO**

FRANKINCENSE: *Boswellia thurifera*
Gum: antiseptic, tonic, astringent, carminative.

FUMITORY: *Fumaria officinalis*
Aerial parts: antispasmodic, liver and gall bladder stimulant.

GAN CAO: *Glycyrrhiza uralensis*
Root: diaphoretic, antirheumatic, analgesic, antispasmodic.

GENTIAN: *Gentiana lutea*
Root: digestive stimulant, sedative, anti-inflammatory, febrifuge.

GINKGO: *Ginkgo biloba*
Leaves: relax blood vessels, circulatory stimulant.

GOAT'S RUE: *Galega officinalis*
Aerial parts: antispasmodic, stimulant. Caution: diabetics should avoid unless under professional guidance.

GOLDEN ROD: *Solidago virgaurea*
Aerial parts: anticatarrhal, diaphoretic, anti-inflammatory, urinary antiseptic, sedative, reduces blood pressure.

GOTU KOLA: *Centella asiatica*
Aerial parts: diuretic, sedating nervine, cooling, tonic. Caution: high doses can cause headaches or aggravate itching.

GOU QI ZI: *Lycium chinense*
Berries: energy tonic, lowers blood pressure, lowers cholesterol.

GRAVELROOT:
Eupatorium purpureum
Root: diuretic, antirheumatic, encourages menstruation.

GROUND IVY: *Glechoma hederacea*
Leaves: astringent, anticatarrhal.

GUARANA: *Paullinia cupana*
Seeds: stimulant, caffeine source.

GUELDER ROSE, CRAMP BARK:
Viburnum opulus
Bark: antispasmodic, sedative, astringent, muscle relaxant, cardiac tonic, uterine relaxant, anti-inflammatory.

HAWTHORN: *Crataegus oxyacantha*
Flowering tops, berries: relaxes blood vessels, cardiac tonic, astringent.

HELONIAS see FALSE UNICORN ROOT

HOPS: *Humulus lupulus*
Strobiles: sedative, male anaphrodisiac, nerve tonic, bitter digestive stimulant, diuretic. Cautions: do not exceed the stated dose. Avoid in depression. The growing plant can cause skin rashes.

HORSETAIL: *Equisetum arvense*
Aerial parts: astringent, stop bleeding, diuretic, anti-inflammatory, tissue healer.

ISPHAGULA, PSYLLIUM SEEDS:
Plantago ovata
Seeds: demulcent, laxative.

JU HUA, CHINESE CHRYSANTHEMUM:
Chrysanthemum morifolium
Flowers: anti-inflammatory, antimicrobial, lower blood pressure.

KELP, BLADDERWRACK:
Fucus vesiculosis
Thalli: metabolic stimulant, thyroid tonic, nutritive, antirheumatic, anti-inflammatory.

LADY'S MANTLE: *Alchemilla vulgaris*
Aerial parts: astringent, menstrual regulator, digestive tonic, anti-inflammatory. Caution: avoid in pregnancy.

LESSER CELANDINE see PILEWORT

LIAN QIAO, FORSYTHIA:
Forsythia suspensa
Fruit: antibacterial, anti-inflammatory, antirheumatic, circulatory stimulant. Caution: avoid in diarrhoea.

LING ZHI: *Ganoderma lucidem*
Fruiting body: immune stimulant, nervine, tonic, anti-tussive, anti-allergenic, anti-bacterial.

LINSEED: *Linum usitatissimum*
Seeds: demulcent, soothing, anti-tussive, antiseptic, anti-inflammatory, laxative. Cautions: Do not drink artists' linseed oil. Do not exceed the stated dose.

LUNGWORT: *Pulmonaria officinalis*
Flowering plant: soothing expectorant, astringent, styptic.

MAGNOLIA see XIN YIN HUA

MA HUANG, EPHEDRA:
Ephedra sinica
Twigs: febrifuge, antispasmodic, diaphoretic, diuretic, antibacterial. Cautions: restricted herb in the UK, for use by professional practitioners only. Restricted herb in Australia and New Zealand. Not to be used if taking MAO inhibitors as antidepressants. Should be avoided in cases of glaucoma, hypertension and coronary thrombosis.

MARJORAM: *Origanum marjorana*
Leaves, essential oil: stimulant, promote menstruation, antispasmodic, diaphoretic.

MILK THISTLE: *Carduus marianus*
Seeds: liver stimulant and tonic, promote milk flow, demulcent, antidepressant.

MOTHERWORT: *Leonurus cardiaca*
Aerial parts: uterine stimulant, relaxant, cardiac tonic, carminative. Caution: avoid in pregnancy; safe in labour.

MUGWORT: *Artemisia vulgaris*
Aerial parts: bitter digestive tonic, stimulant, stimulating nervine, menstrual regulator, antirheumatic. Cautions: avoid in pregnancy and if breastfeeding.

MULLEIN: *Verbascum thapsus*
Flowers, leaves: expectorant, mild diuretic, demulcent, sedative, heal wounds, astringent, anti-inflammatory.

MYRRH: *Commiphora molmol*
Resin, essential oil: antifungal, antiseptic, astringent, bitter, expectorant, circulatory stimulant, anticatarrhal. Caution: avoid in pregnancy.

NUTMEG: *Myristica fragrans*
Kernel, essential oil: carminative, digestive stimulant, antispasmodic, prevents vomiting, appetite stimulant, anti-inflammatory. Cautions: large doses (7.5 g or more in a single dose) are dangerous, producing convulsions and palpitations. Avoid in pregnancy.

NU ZHEN ZI: *Ligustrum lucidum*
Berries: tonic, immunostimulant, diuretic.

OATS: *Avena sativa*
Grain: antidepressant, restorative nerve tonic, nutritive. Oatbran: anti-thrombotic, reduces blood cholesterol levels. Caution: those sensitive to gluten must allow the decoction or tincture to settle, then decant the clear liquid only for use.

PAPAYA: *Carica papaya*
Fruit: rich in vitamins, digestive remedy, anti-allergenic, wound herb.

PASSIONFLOWER: *Passiflora incarnata*
Leaves: sedative, anodyne, hypnotic, antispasmodic. Caution: avoid high doses in pregnancy.

PATCHOULI: *Pogostemon cablin*
Essential oil: antidepressant, aphrodisiac, sedative, tonic, antiseptic.

PELLITORY-OF-THE-WALL:
Parietaria diffusa
Aerial parts: demulcent, diuretic.

PILEWORT, LESSER CELANDINE:
Ranunculus ficaria
Root, leaves: astringent.

PINE: *Pinus sylvestris*
Essential oil: expectorant, antiseptic, decongestant, rubefacient.

PLEURISY ROOT: *Asclepias tuberosa*
Root: expectorant, carminative, laxative, relaxes peripheral blood vessels.

PRICKLY ASH:
Zanthoxylum americanum
Bark: carminative, circulatory stimulant, promotes sweating, tonic.

PSYLLIUM SEEDS see ISPHAGULA

RAMSOMS: *Allium ursinum*
Aerial parts, bulbs: decrease blood sugar levels, lower cholesterol, antimicrobial.

RASPBERRY: *Rubus idaeus*
Leaves: astringent, preparative for childbirth, stimulant, digestive tonic. Berries: diuretic, laxative, diaphoretic, cleansing. Caution: avoid high doses of the leaves during early pregnancy.

RED CLOVER: *Trifolium pratense*
Flowers: cleansing, antispasmodic, diuretic, anti-inflammatory, possible oestrogenic activity.

RHUBARB: *Rheum palmatum*
Root: laxative, digestive tonic, astringent, antibacterial. Cautions: avoid in pregnancy, gout and arthritic conditions. The leaves are toxic.

ROSE: *Rosa* spp
Essential oil: antidepressant, antispasmodic, sedative, aphrodisiac, cleansing, expectorant, antibacterial, antiviral, antiseptic, kidney tonic, blood tonic, menstrual regulator, anti-inflammatory. Cautions: only use the best quality oil medicinally. Only take internally under professional supervision.

SANDALWOOD: *Santalum album*
Essential oil: antidepressant, antiseptic, antispasmodic, carminative, expectorant.

SAW PALMETTO: *Serenoa repens*
Berries: aphrodisiac, diuretic, sedative.

SELF-HEAL: *Prunella vulgaris*
Aerial parts: antibacterial, reduce blood pressure, diuretic, astringent, heal wounds. **Flower spikes:** liver stimulant, reduce blood pressure, antibacterial.

SENNA: *Cassia senna*
Leaves, fruits: stimulating, laxative. **Caution:** avoid in pregnancy, unless prescribed by professional practitioner.

SHU DI HUANG:
Rehmannia glutinosa
Prepared root: demulcent, laxative, styptic, blood tonic.

SLIPPERY ELM: *Ulmus fulva*
Bark: demulcent, nutritive, astringent.

SOAP BARK: *Quillaja saponaria*
Inner bark: detergent, expectorant,

anti-inflammatory. **Caution:** do not take internally.

SUNDEW: *Drosera rotundifolia*
Flowering plant: relaxant expectorant, antispasmodic, demulcent.

SWEET SUMACH: *Rhus aromatica*
Root, bark: astringent, diuretic, antidiabetic.

TEA: *Camellia sinensis*
Leaves: stimulant, astringent, antibacterial, diuretic.

THUJA: *Thuja occidentalis*
Leaf tips: astringent, antimicrobial, anti-inflammatory, muscle stimulant. **Caution:** avoid in pregnancy.

TORMENTIL: *Potentilla erecta*
Root: astringent.

UVA-URSI *see* **BEARBERRY**

VALERIAN: *Valeriana officinalis*
Root: tranquillizing, antispasmodic,

expectorant, diuretic, reduces blood pressure, carminative, mild anodyne. **Cautions:** do not take for more than 2–3 weeks without a break. Avoid if taking sleep-inducing drugs.

WHITE DEADNETTLE:
Lamium album
Flowering tops: astringent, tonic for reproductive organs, antispasmodic.

WHITE HOREHOUND:
Marrubium vulgare
Aerial parts: antispasmodic, bitter, stimulating expectorant, soothing tonic.

WHITE PAEONY *see* **BAI SHAO**

WILD CHERRY: *Prunus serotina*
Bark: anti-tussive, digestive stimulant, sedative. **Cautions:** avoid in acute infections. Can cause drowsiness.

WILLOW: *Salix alba*
Bark, leaves: antirheumatic, anti-

septic, anti-inflammatory, analgesic, astringent, bitter digestive tonic.

WITCH HAZEL:
Hamamelis virginiana
Bark, leaves: astringent, haemostatic. **Cautions:** use externally only.

WORMWOOD: *Artemesia absinthium*
Aerial parts: bitter digestive tonic, uterine stimulant, antibiotic, bile stimulant, carminative, antiseptic. **Caution:** avoid if pregnant or breastfeeding.

XIN YIN HUA, MAGNOLIA:
Magnolia liliflora
Flower, flowerbuds: anticatarrhal, antifungal, analgesic, anti-inflammatory. **Cautions:** high doses can cause dizziness.

YLANG YLANG: *Cananga odorata*
Essential oil: antidepressant, antiseptic, aphrodisiac, sedative. **Caution:** use sparingly, excess can cause headaches and nausea.

Glossary

Analgesic: relieves pain.
Anodyne: allays pain.
Antispasmodic: reduces muscle spasm and tension.
Anti-tussive: inhibits coughing reflex.
Aperient: mild laxative.
Bitter: stimulates secretion of digestive juices, stimulates appetite.
Carminative: relieves flatulence and digestive colic.
Demulcent: soothes damaged or inflamed surfaces.
Diaphoretic: promotes sweating.
Diuretic: encourages urine flow.
Febrifuge: reduces fever.
Mucilage: soft, slippery substances that protect mucous membranes.
Nervine: affects the nervous system.
Rubefacient: stimulates blood flow to the skin.
Saponins: plant substance similar to soap; expectorant.
Styptic: stops external bleeding.
Systemic: affecting the entire body.
Tonify: strengthen and restore.
Topical: local adminstration of a remedy, e.g. to the skin.
Yang: associated with male energy – dry, hot.
Yin: associated with female energy – damp, cold.

Consulting a Herbalist & Addresses

In the UK, there are two main professional bodies: The National Institute of Medical Herbalists and The General Council and Register of Consultant Herbalists. There is also The Register of Traditional Chinese Medicine, whose members practise a combination of acupuncture and Chinese herbalism.

Herbalists vary in their approach. Some, for example, use a combination of therapies, such as naturopathy and massage as well as prescribing remedies. Choose your practitioner by personal recommendation if possible, otherwise ask the herbalist about his or her approach before making an appointment.

A first consultation will last about an hour, during which time the practitioner will take a case history, do some clinical tests (e.g. take blood pressure) and make any relevant physical examinations. At the end, he or she will dispense the remedy in the form of tinctures, dried herbs, capsules, creams, etc., and give advice on diet and lifestyle.

KEY
• postal supplier (mail order)
* retail supplier

British Herbal Medicine Association
Sun House, Church Street, Stroud, Gloucestershire GL5 1JL
The General Council and Register of Consultant Herbalists
Marlborough House, Swanpool, Falmouth, Cornwall TR11 4HW
The Herb Society
134 Buckingham Palace Road, London SW1W 9SA
National Institute of Medical Herbalists
56 Longbrook Street, Exeter, Devon EX4 6AH
The Natural Medicines Group Secretariat
PO Box 5, Ilkeston, Derbyshire DE7 8LX
The Register of Chinese Herbal Medicine
98b Hazelville Road, London N19 3NA.

Herbal Suppliers
• * Baldwin, G. & Co., 171–173 Walworth Road, London SE17 1RW
* Culpeper Ltd (Head Office) Hadstock Road, Linton Cambridge CB1 2NJ
• East West Herbs Ltd Langston Priory Mews, Kingham, Oxon OX7 6UW

* East West Herbs Shop 2 Neal's Yard, Covent Garden, London WC2E 9DP
• Gerard House 3 Wickham Road, Boscomb, Bournemouth BH7 6JX
• The Herbal Apothecary 120 High Street, Syston, Leics IE7 8GC
* Napier & Sons 18 Nicholson Street, Edinburgh, Eh8 9DJ
* Neal's Yard Remedies (Head Office) 1a Rossiter Road, London SW12 9RY
• Potters Herbal Supplies Leyland Mill Lane, Wigan, Lancs WN1 2SB

Equipment suppliers
Most of the equipment needed can be bought from good chemists (e.g. anhydrous lanolin, glycerine, cocoa butter, bottles, jars) or from wine-making specialists or department stores (wine presses, jelly bags, etc.).
• Dav-Caps PO Box 48, Hitchin, Herts SG4 9BT (*Capsules and capsule-making machines*)
• Quaestus The Sudio, Llanbedr, Crickhowell, Powys, Wales NP8 1SR (*Pessary moulds*)

INDEX

NOTE: Page numbers in **bold** refer to main herb entries in the *A-to-Z of Medicinal Herbs* and *Other Medicinal Herbs*.

Author's Acknowledgments

Like enthusiastic cooks, medical herbalists endlessly collect and
adapt ideas for using herbs, as well as "recipes" for creams,
syrups or lotions, from friends and colleagues. My thanks are
therefore due to many fellow herbalists who have generously
shared their knowledge with me over very many years. It
would be impossible to list everyone – it may read like the
membership roll of the NIMH – but especial love and
gratitude to Andrew Chevallier, Stephen and Carol Church,
Carole Guyett, Christopher Hedley, Rowan Stainton, Dragana
Carter and Anne Warren-Davis.

Publisher's Acknowledgments

Dorling Kindersley would like to thank: Peter Allen (*Ugly*
modelling agency), Jane, Stephen, Charlotte and William Bull,
Thomas Greene, Mary Ody, Hossein Razazan, Nicki Sarluis,
Kate Scott, Susan Swaris and Tina Vaughan for modelling;
Ellen Cramer (*Artistic Licence* agency) for make up; Stephen
Bull for collecting herb specimens; Rosemary Titterington at
Iden Croft Herbs and Chelsea Physic Garden; Helen Barnett,
Antonia Cunningham, Charlotte Evans, Nell Graville, Valerie
Horn, Colin Nicholls and Nick Turpin for editorial assistance;
and Sarah Ereira for compiling the index.

Photography Credits

key to picture positions: t=top b=bottom r=right l=left c=centre

All photography by Steve Gorton except:
Peter Anderson: 40 tr; 44 bc, br. Martin Cameron: 55; 56 (tl, tr, br);
57; 63 bl, br; 68 (except tr); 70 t,l; 71 tl, tr, bl, br; 72 (except tr); 73 (except
tl); 75 bl; 76 bl, br. Andy Crawford: 53 b, r; 63 tc, tr; 66-7; 68 tr; 69 br;
70 b; 71 bc; 72 tr; 74; 75 (except bl); 76 tl, tc, tr; 77; 78-9. Nigel Fletcher
and Matthew Ward: 20 t; 31 tr; 33 bl; 34 c; 35 tr; 36 bc; 39 br; 46 bl; 95 bl.
Dave King: 2-3; 5 tl, br; 8-9; 10 bl-br; 12 b (except br); 14 bl-br; 16 bl-br;
17; 18 b (except left oil); 20 b (except br); 22 b (except br); 24 bl-br;
26 bl-br; 28-9; 37 tc; 39 tl; 40 br, bc; 41 br; 42 c; 43 r; 48-9; 52
(except widger); 56 bl; 58-9; 62; 64-5; 80-1; 82-3; 84-5; 102-3 tc; 145.
David Murray: 38 l. National Trust Photographic Library/Mike Williams:
50. Martin Norris: 136 tl, tc. Tim Ridley: 12 br; 18 bc (oil); 20 br, 22 br.
Steve Shott: 11. Clive Streeter: 31 bl; 33 tl; 43 tl; 60-1; 86; 88; 92-3; 103
(dried bistort root); 104-5; 106-7; 111; 134; 135 t, cr, br.
Matthew Ward: 115 lc.

The Herb Society

The Herb Society was founded by Hilda Leyel in 1927 as the Society of
Herbalists: the society sold culinary, medicinal and cosmetic herbs and
products. Having "always experimented in the innocent alchemy of scent
blending and cooking" Mrs Leyel dedicated herself to research into
herbal medicine from 1926. Today, The Herb Society has an international
membership which includes professional growers, historians, medical
herbalists, amateur gardeners, beauticians and cooks. It publishes *Herbs*,
the UK's only specialist magazine devoted to all aspects of herbs, and a
newsletter, *Herbarium*, which provides information on the latest
research, herb books, overseas publications, and membership activities.
Regular seminars and workshops are arranged worldwide. The Herb
Society Garden, which incorporates Apothecaries' Paradise and Knot
Gardens is part of the Henry Doubleday Research Association's Yalding
Gardens in Kent. The Society provides specialist answers to members'
queries and information on herb courses, herb gardens, sources, literature
and local herb groups. See p. 140 for address.   040-602-1